Sweet Tea & Cornbread

Inspiring, Motivating & Empowering
Black Women to Take Back Their Bodies &
Live a Healthier Lifestyle

Karrie Marchbanks

This book is intended to supplement, not replace, the advice of a trained health professional. If you know or suspect you have a health problem, you should consult a health professional. The author and publisher specifically disclaim any liability, loss or risk, personal or otherwise, that is incurred as a consequence, directly or indirectly, of the use or application of any of the contents of this book.

10 9 8 7 6 5 4 3 2 1

Published in the United States of America

ISBN-13: 978-1478233039
ISBN-10: 1478233036

DEDICATION

To all the phenomenal women in my life.
You nurtured me, raised me, disciplined me, cared for me,
shared with me, protected me, inspired me, prayed with me,
prayed for me, encouraged me, mentored me, cried with me,
listened to me, fought for me, fought beside me, motivated me...
and loved me.
I am because you are.

"It wasn't until I actually did have my own place that I realized how certain memories tuck themselves away, deep in the recesses of your mind and don't come out until one day you're sitting on the couch, in your pajamas, with a mixing bowl full of cereal."

- KM

Contents

How to Use This Book

Welcome to the revolution! <u>Sweet Tea and Cornbread</u> is a combination of humorous stories, health information and action plans designed to encourage, inspire and educate black women to better health!

There are 21 chapters and 21 Affirmation pages in this book. Each chapter represents one day. Read one chapter per day starting with Day 1. After you have read the chapter, complete the Affirmation page. The Affirmation pages are designed to help you put into action what you have just learned, reconnect you to the woman you are inside and help you bring insight to those things that might be holding you back from living the life you deserve. If you feel as though you need more writing space or you're reading an eBook, it's perfectly fine to use a spiral notebook as a daily journal. The important thing is to take your time in answering the questions, put some thought into it and be honest with yourself. The more open and honest you are, the more life changing and real the work becomes.

For those of you who learn better by doing, read one chapter per week for 21 weeks. Start on a Sunday, read Day 1, complete the Affirmation page and use the rest of the week to implement what you've just learned. The following Sunday read Day 2 and so on until you've completed the entire book.

I am so excited that you've made the decision to take control of your body and live a healthier lifestyle! Get your highlighters ready because this book is packed with useful information you will want to go back to time and time again. Today is the first day of the rest of your life and together we're going to make sure it's a long, healthy life!

Introduction

If you're like me, you sometimes reminisce about the good ole days, the pre-gravity days or PGD as I like to call them. The days when you could eat whatever you wanted, you didn't have to exercise, and all your body parts looked exactly the way God intended. Thighs didn't rub together, boobs didn't sag, and a muffin top was something you ate, preferably warm with butter. Remember? You know what I'm talking about, right? Like when you looked down at your feet, not only could you see them, you could actually touch them on command! And when you waved goodbye there was no breeze created by the flapping of saggy arms. Back fat was something other people had instead of something you now have three remedies for and a dozen outfits to disguise. You were a glowing representation of youthful perfection. So what happened? Was it age? Your love of fast food? Heredity? Or do you let your emotions tell you it's okay to eat a carton of ice cream, as long as you save a little for tomorrow? <u>Sweet Tea and Cornbread</u> was written for every black woman who identifies with the struggle to eat healthy, lose weight and exercise just enough to see results but not enough to sweat out a fresh relaxer. With chapters like *Maybe You're Not Just Big Boned* and *Red, Purple and Orange are Colors, Not Drinks!* you will laugh as you discover why your body responds to sugar the way it does and learn the most effective ways to exercise for your body type. Each chapter is filled with information from a cultural point of view and designed to teach you how to eat in the real world without mail order food or expensive diet plans. Sweet Tea and Cornbread will inspire, encourage and motivate you to take back your body and live a healthier lifestyle.

Let's face it ladies, as black women we have issues when it comes to food and exercise -- issues that are unique to us as African Americans. I had a Great-Aunt who used to say "black folks eat everything from the rooter to the tooter!" Meaning as far as a pig was concerned, nothing went to waste; you ate the whole pig front to back! In her day they transformed scraps into meals fit for a king. Today we call it *soul food* and unfortunately, the culinary masterpieces we've handed down from generation to generation are, in part, responsible for our ever increasing dress sizes and high risk for chronic disease. Soul food is typically high in fat, sodium and sugar, but I'm going to show you in chapters like ***Grandma Did It, Mama Did It, I'll Do It*** how to make substitutions in your favorite recipes so you can continue to eat the foods you love, but in a healthier way.

When it comes to exercise, there's not a black woman in America who won't identify with the chapter entitled ***Do What? I Just Got My Hair Done!*** because we were taught at an early age that water in any form whether it be perspiration, rain, sleet or snow and a black woman's hair, don't mix! Regularly scheduled exercise is something most black women stopped doing after junior high school. It wasn't fun, it made your body hurt, and if you're never going to be in the Olympics or play professional sports what's the point, right? Wrong! The reality is black women lead the country in every chronic disease. I'm talking about high blood pressure, high cholesterol, diabetes, heart disease and obesity and the only way we're going to lose that title is to change our eating habits and exercise more.

Incorporating exercise into your daily routine doesn't mean you have to give up your weave in favor of something more natural, nor does it mean you have to pump iron till you look like a man. As black women, we've let our hairstyles determine the size of our waistlines, and it's killing us! Pride in your appearance shouldn't stop at the neck. The American Heart Association reports that **38.8% or two out of five black women in America have more than one chronic disease.** Two out of five! How does the Pastor say it at church? Look to your right and then to your left, if you're not the one with chronic disease, both of the people sitting next to you are. In the chapter, **I Used to Run Every Day. Now My Knees Hurt so Bad I Can't** I share my own personal story about my struggle to lose weight and how denial kept me overweight for years.

Sweet Tea and Cornbread is the literary manifestation of my passion to help women be successful in all areas of their life, starting with their health. Take control of this area and you'll have the energy, strength, confidence and courage to take control in other areas of your life as well. How do I know this? I'm not a doctor nor do I have my own TV show; I'm just a black woman who has fought the good fight and won! I've battled through divorce, single parenting, financial difficulties and weight issues, just like you. I've spent hundreds on exercise equipment and videos just like you, drank diet shakes till I had enough gas in my stomach to power a Prius, just like you. I was broke, busted and disgusted! Nothing worked and then one day I looked in the mirror, didn't recognize myself and said, "ENOUGH!" I set out on a mission to understand why my body was betraying me, and while on that mission, I realized that not only was I responsible for the shape my body was in, I was sabotaging every effort I had made to lose weight for two reasons; first, I didn't understand the basics of nutrition and second, I didn't understand the relationship between nutrition and the black community. For black women, our inability to lose weight is more than just a hand-to-mouth thing; it's also a black thing. The way we view food, what we eat and the way we eat it goes back to slavery times and until we modernize our thinking and understand the health risks we face because of it, black women will continue to be overweight, undernourished and continue to suffer disproportionately from chronic disease. I wrote this book to help you understand the relationship between our culture, food and how our bodies respond to exercise so that you'll have the tools you need to drop the word <u>diet</u> from your vocabulary forever and take control of your body once and for all.

No, the revolution won't be televised, but the results will be felt for years to come in the health of our families and our children's families. Today is the day black women say <u>no</u> to chronic disease and say <u>yes</u> to living a healthier lifestyle. Today is the day we say no to the stereotypical images of black women and the media's perception of what beauty is. Today is the day you look in the mirror and see yourself for who you truly are – a phenomenal black woman, fearfully and wonderfully made in God's image with the power and skill to do all things, in Jesus' name, AMEN!

Day 1
Maybe You're Not Just Big Boned

I don't know where it came from or how it started, but I can remember when I was a little girl hearing people say, "Oh, he's not fat, he's just big boned," or "All the women in my family are big boned." I grew up believing that, for reasons beyond the parameters of my childhood mind, God created some people with extra thick bones. Bones so thick the person actually looked fat! Truth be told, I had a few "big boned" people in my family. Cousin Betty, with her fly afro, hot pink coulats (capri's for the younger generation) and flowered halter top didn't mind parading her big bones for all to see at family picnics. Or how about Uncle Junebug, who looked more like Santa Claus (in his white undershirt, stomach hanging out) than a Junebug. I learned to equate being overweight with a God-given condition that no one could do anything about. Some people had it, and some people didn't; it was that simple.

Unfortunately, the "big boned" myth rears its ugly head at family picnics and family reunions to this day. Jokingly or not, you hear the term said in movies, comedy routines, at work, at home and among friends. The idea that some people have big bones, and not a hand-to-mouth problem has been a joke and an excuse in the black community for years. So let me clear this up right now! Your skeleton is absolutely, 100% unique to you, and although you *can* have a small, medium or large skeletal frame, the size of your bones has nothing to do with the circumference of your waistline or how "thick" your thighs are. If you drank nothing but water for three weeks you would probably lose a few pounds, but your bones would still be the same size. You can eat

1

all the cakes, pies and ice cream your heart desires and your bones will not grow any larger. You could have a meat fest and eat ribs, chicken, goat, rabbit, gator or coon till you're about to explode and guess what, you'll still have the same size bones. Get the point? Can we move on? Great!

So, if there's no such thing as being "big boned," what's the problem? I'm so glad you asked! The answer starts with determining your body type. There are three body types: Endomorph (fat retainers), Mesomorph (athletic physique - we hate you!), and Ectomorph (skinny - we hate you more!).

> **Endomorphs** have a soft, curvy or round physique. They have a low metabolic rate, gain weight easily and have to work hard to keep the pounds off. They usually have a pear-shaped physique meaning fat settles in the lower abdomen, hips, butt and thighs. This shape has a lower risk of developing heart disease caused by obesity. But, if they have a round physique, fat accumulates in the abdomen, arms, and legs which puts them at greater risk for heart disease, diabetes and other chronic diseases. Famous endomorphs include; Oprah, Queen Latifah, Beyonce, Monique, and Mary J. Blige.

> **Mesomorphs** are naturally lean, muscular and strong. They usually have broad shoulders which create an hourglass figure in women. Their metabolic rate is efficient, and their bodies respond well to exercise so it's easy for them to gain muscle and lose fat. They are natural born athletes. Think First Lady Michelle Obama, Serena Williams, Angela Bassett, Tina Turner, or Halle Berry.

> **Ectomorphs** are slim, have long arms and legs and have very little body fat or muscle. They are small in the shoulder and hip area giving them a long, lean look. It seems as though they can eat anything they want and

never gain a pound because their metabolic rate is so high. However, gaining muscle bulk can be a challenge for them. Basketball players, ballerina's and most high fashion models fall into this category. Famous ectomorphs include; Whitney Houston, Naomi Campbell, Kelly Rowland, and Cicely Tyson. [1]

Now, I'm not going to ask you to get naked and stand in front of a full length mirror, you know all too well where your body collects its fat and if you are over 40 it is probably collecting it in places you never thought possible. As we age our bodies can morph from one type to another. When I was a teenager my body type was ectomorphic. I was an athlete and couldn't gain a pound. My grandmother would push food at me like she was on suicide watch! "Don't you want another piece of cake?" she would say, and I was more than happy to oblige. I always got seconds and received many a dirty look from my endomorphic cousins. After college and after giving birth to my daughter, the weight I gained settled in my hips and thighs. Now for me that was a good thing; I finally had some curves! But that pear can quickly turn into an apple if you don't watch out. Thank the Lord for making me tall because now at the age of 48 it's harder than ever to maintain my endomorphic body. I'm still a pear, maybe more of a dinner pear than a snack pear, but a pear nevertheless!

It's no secret that in order to lose weight or maintain a healthy weight you have to eat less and move more. Duh, right? Well, for most of us that common sense goes right out the window when we drive by Krispy Kreme and see the "Hot" light shining in the window. Tell me, how many times have you pulled up to the drive through window and answered, "small" to the question, "would you like that small, medium or large?" And I know you *always* leave the second bag or box of (insert your favorite junk food here) at the store when its buy one get one free. Right?

If knowing your body type is the first step, then understanding how to exercise that body type is the next.

Endomorphs have a higher body fat percentage. So, as an endomorph your primary focus should be on cardiovascular exercise *and* fat burning. Endomorphs should either start weight training immediately or wait until you have reached a weight with which you are more happy.

The advantage of waiting is that once you have lost weight you'll have a better idea of how much weight training you need to do. You will also be able to see a greater change in terms of weight loss and inches lost. On the other hand, starting your weight training regimen immediately allows you to ensure that you are not losing muscle mass, as often occurs with dieting. Remember, muscle burns calories. The key for endomorphs to achieve a good physique is dropping fat and preserving muscle.

Mesomorphs should focus on weight loss to shrink your waistline. The best exercise for you is cardio, simply shaping and contouring the curves of your figure. The goal is to create a lot of shape. Mesomorphs should concentrate on a strong cardio workout (aerobics, treadmill, elliptical) and limit weights. If you're worried about overly muscular legs you can do exercises that will slim down your calves or slim down thighs (running works great). With regular exercising, this body type tends to sculpt and shape well-defined muscles more easily than ectomorphs or endomorphs.

Ectomorphs need to stimulate their muscles deeply in order to increase their muscle mass. An ectomorph has to start their workout with a well thought out plan. You need to work intensely with heavy weights and low repetitions. Avoid isolation exercises, which only target individual muscles. This tactic won't achieve the kind of full body muscle stimulation you require. Instead, go for major compound exercises such as the bench press, squats, dead lifts or lunges. Also, exercises using barbells and dumbbells are great, as they allow you to use full range of motion. The more muscles you work, the more muscle growth you get. [1]

Okay ladies, time for a test. The next time you hear somebody say they're "big boned" what are you going to say? "There's no such thing as a big boned person, you're an endomorph!" I'm so proud of you I could cry! We know that Cousin Betty and Uncle Junebug weren't big boned; they were just plain fat! They may have started out as ectomorphs or mesomorphs, but they became endomorphs! And we know that with a little less hand-to-mouth action and a lot more exercise they could have changed all that. WE can change all that! Today is the first day on your quest to living a healthier life style. Let the revolution begin!

Today's Challenge

Today I challenge you to embrace your body type and fall in love with the person you are inside of it -- the person God created. Believe with all your heart that you deserve the very best life has to offer and make a commitment to yourself right now that you will do whatever it takes to have it. Let nothing stand in your way, especially your health.

Day 1 Affirmation

"Hear, O LORD, and be merciful to me; O LORD, be my help. You turned my wailing into dancing; you removed my sackcloth and clothed me with joy, that my heart may sing to you and not be silent. O LORD my God, I will give you thanks forever."

Psalm 30:10-12

WHAT DID YOU LEARN FROM TODAY'S READING AND WHAT DID YOU LEARN ABOUT YOURSELF?

_____
_____
_____
_____
_____
_____
_____
_____
_____
_____
_____
_____

HOW WILL YOU TAKE ONE STEP TOWARDS LIVING A HEALTHIER LIFESTYLE TODAY?

_____
_____
_____
_____
_____
_____
_____
_____
_____
_____
_____
_____

LIST THREE THINGS (ANY THING)YOU'RE PROUD OF YOURSELF FOR TODAY AND EXPLAIN WHY:

_____

_____

_____

_____

_____

_____

_____

_____

_____

_____

_____

_____

_____

_____

_____

SPEND FIVE MINUTES TODAY RECONNECTING YOUR SPIRIT TO GOD. WRITE IT, PRAY IT OR SHOW IT!

_____

_____

_____

_____

_____

_____

_____

_____

_____

_____

_____

_____

_____

_____

_____

_____

Day 2
I Eat What I Want, That's What the Pills are For

"Are you serious?!" That's exactly what I said to my friend as we sat in a restaurant and I watched her order and eat a huge chicken breast smothered with brown gravy, sitting atop a bed of white rice. No vegetables, instead she had a salad with Ranch dressing and breadsticks. Oh, I forgot to mention the New York style cheesecake she ordered to go! "I'm not gonna eat it now. I'll be craving something sweet later," she said with a smile. Now I know what you're thinking, "Let the girl eat!" Right? And some of you have already made a mental note to have that for dinner tonight. Well go ahead with your bad selves! That's what the pills are for, aren't they?

You see, my friend, like so many black women in America, is overweight, has high cholesterol and diabetes. I wasn't just trying to stop her from enjoying a meal; I was trying to save her life! You have to understand, this wasn't the first time all the "Girlz" (a moniker we came up with to represent our group) had gathered together for dinner. We do it on the regular; it's our way of staying connected. Once a month we'll meet for lunch, dinner or go away for the weekend. We've gone to the beach, the mountains, taken cruises, seen concerts and plays together. We talk about our jobs, love lives, current events, which male actor is our fantasy love interest (Idris Elba! Can I get an Amen!), the kids and grandkids. You know how women do, no topic is off limits. We've been meeting like this for over 10 years, so when I asked her if she was serious about eating that particular meal; it was with genuine love and concern.

I've watched my friends grow over the years mentally, spiritually and *physically,* and I've watched their health decline in the process! We were at dinner one night, and the topic of conversation switched to medication. It was weird for me to sit there and listen to them talk about which medication they were on and for what ailment. One of them said, "Girl, tell your doctor to put you on this pill, it doesn't make your feet swell up!" Another chimed in, "My doctor put me on a new cholesterol pill and now I can't stop going to the bathroom." Still another said, "I just eat what I want, check my sugar and give myself a shot." I held up my hand in an attempt to stop the conversation and said, "Ladies, are we really going to spend the night talking about what medications we're on?" They all laughed, and someone made the comment, "I guess that's what happens when you get old." Old? This is what happens when you get old? Now, in my mind I'm thinking old is somewhere around 80 and even that will be debatable when I get there! Our ages range from 40 to 60, and I'm the only one in the group who is not taking medication for some type of chronic disease. Unfortunately, the demographics of our little group appear to match up with the health statistics for black women in America as a whole.

Here's how black women rate when it comes to chronic disease.*

- 47.3% have cardiovascular disease.
- 45.7% have high blood pressure.
- 41.2% have high cholesterol.
- 51.0% are obese (BMI of 30.0kg/m^2 or higher)
- 14.7% have diabetes
- 38.8% have metabolic syndrome (having more than one chronic disease)

*American Heart Association Statistical Fact Sheet Update 2012

Need I go on? The numbers are staggering, downright scary if you think about it! With statistics like that, you would think there would be a mind boggling revolution among black women to eat healthier and exercise more. Instead, we take a pill. We give ourselves a shot. The legacy we're leaving for our daughters is one of poor health and disease, and they deserve better than that. The chronic diseases mentioned here are all PREVENTABLE if you are not genetically predisposed to contracting them and even if you are, your goal should still be to live a healthier lifestyle. You have the ability to change the condition of your health today, this instant! So why don't we do it?

I've asked my group of friends and relatives this exact question and the answers are as varied as they are. I've heard them say things like, "It's too expensive to eat healthy." Or, "I don't have time to eat healthy." And, "I could get hit by a car tomorrow; I'm going to enjoy myself!" Oh and I love this one, "My kids won't eat healthy stuff." Ok, say it with me, "Are you serious?!" Let's examine these responses for any shred of sanity.

1. "It's too expensive to eat healthy." – Which usually translates into, "I don't feel like cooking." So let's compare apples to apples so to speak. A grilled chicken salad and drink from a typical drive thru costs about $7.00. Purchase a bag of organic lettuce, two tomatoes, a cucumber, and pre-packaged grilled chicken from your local grocery store and spend around $10.32. What? You thought the cost was going to be less? I'm not a magician, but don't miss the point. By making your own salad the meal is healthier and instead of feeding yourself for the day, you've just purchased enough food for lunch for three days. $10.32 divided by 3 equals $3.44 a day and you'll save on gas too!

2. "I don't have time to eat healthy!" – Which usually means you're pulling up to the drive through window three times a day. Not only is eating out expensive, if you don't watch the foods you choose you'll quickly put on the pounds. Convenience is the mother of obesity! Fast food is typically high in fat, salt and sugar and we know what that does to our bodies. So what can you do? God created the perfect on-the-go foods; they're called fruits, nuts and vegetables! Pack your favorite fruits and raw vegetables, along with nuts and whole grain crackers, and you've got lunch or healthy snacks that curb your appetite and give you the nutrition your body needs. For example, I would rather sleep than get up early to cook breakfast before I go to work, so my on-the-go breakfast consists of a peanut butter sandwich (on whole grain, sugar free bread) a banana and soy milk. It's quick, nutritious, and I can eat it in the car. For lunch, I'll pack low sodium, vegetable soup or oatmeal, two kinds of fruit, yogurt, nuts and whole grain crackers. If I don't have time to heat the soup I still have nutritious, fiber rich foods to eat so I'm not tempted to run to the vending machine.

3. "I could get hit by a car tomorrow; I'm going to enjoy myself!" – You know, the bad thing about chronic disease is that it doesn't happen overnight. You don't eat a piece of cake and wake up with high blood pressure. If it did, we would all be more motivated to eat healthier and exercise more. Chronic disease happens over time, and if you don't watch what you eat now you'll wake up one day, look in the mirror and ask yourself what happened? God made our bodies perfect; *we* mess them up! You're kidding yourself if you think chronic disease can't happen to you. I have a cousin who is 37 years old and prides herself on the fact that she eats what she wants, when she

wants. How long do you think it will be before the 30 pounds she's gained turn into 40 and her doctor tells her she's prediabetic? I'm all in favor of living each day to the fullest, but you only have one body and chronic disease is a time bomb. Is the clock ticking for you?

4. "My kids won't eat healthy stuff." – Really?! So essentially your kids run the household, is that what you're telling me? Do your kids work a full-time job, pay the bills and buy the groceries? First of all (and then I'll stop preaching) it's your responsibility to raise your children. The bible says, *"Train up a child in the way he should go, even when he is old he will not depart from it."-Proverbs 22:6.* News flash! That includes teaching them how to eat healthy. Do that and they will teach their children and so on and so on. Babies don't know what anything tastes like until you introduce them to it, so if you feed them sugary or salty foods they develop a craving for it. Have you ever been at a restaurant and ordered sweet tea? If the server brings you unsweetened tea you're ready to fight somebody! Why, because you've developed a "taste" for the sugar in sweet tea and it's hard to change. Some people experience physical withdrawal symptoms when they remove sugar from their diets. I made the decision to raise my daughter sugar and salt free for the first 5 years of her life, and then monitored the amount of processed sugar and salt in her diet by what I bought at the store. *You* decide what food comes into your house; don't sabotage your children's future by giving in to their cries for the latest junk food. The most influential role model your children have is YOU. What are you teaching them about food?

I think it's easy to see the insanity of these comments. The only thing that's holding you back from living a healthier lifestyle is YOU! So I have some questions for you. Where do you see yourself in this story? How many medications are you on? How many times have you eaten too much of the wrong thing, thinking you could fix any adverse effects with a pill or shot? How many people in your family have to die of chronic disease before you hear the wakeup call? **The number one killer of black women over the age of 20 is heart disease. WAKE UP!**

Today's Challenge

Today I challenge you to make a commitment to be an example of good health not only for yourself, but for your family as well. Today is the day you let go of negative thinking and speak life into your decision to live a healthier lifestyle, because whether you think you can or think you can't, you're right! Check your cabinets and refrigerator, right now, and see where you can make changes that will impact your health today.

Day 2 Affirmation

God give me the serenity to accept the things I cannot change, the strength to change the things I can and the wisdom to know the difference.

WHAT DID YOU LEARN FROM TODAY'S READING AND WHAT DID YOU LEARN ABOUT YOURSELF?

_____
_____
_____
_____
_____
_____
_____
_____
_____
_____
_____
_____
_____

HOW WILL YOU TAKE ONE STEP TOWARDS LIVING A HEALTHIER LIFESTYLE TODAY?

_____
_____
_____
_____
_____
_____
_____
_____
_____
_____
_____
_____

LIST THREE THINGS (ANY THING) YOU'RE PROUD OF
YOURSELF FOR TODAY AND EXPLAIN WHY:

_____
_____
_____
_____
_____
_____
_____
_____
_____
_____
_____
_____
_____
_____
_____
_____
_____
_____

SPEND FIVE MINUTES TODAY RECONNECTING YOUR
SPIRIT TO GOD. WRITE IT, PRAY IT OR SHOW IT!

_____
_____
_____
_____
_____
_____
_____
_____
_____
_____
_____
_____
_____
_____
_____
_____

Day 3
Salt is a Condiment, Not a Side Dish

"Baby, what are you doing?" I asked my daughter as I watched her shake salt on the beautiful fresh vegetables I'd just prepared. "They need more salt, they taste…" "What? Fresh?! How do you know they need more, you haven't even tasted them?!" I replied. "Because they always need more salt!" she answered as if to say, "Duh!" All the work I had put into raising my daughter sugar and salt free had gone right out the window as soon as she started high school. Bombarded with hormones, peer pressure and the cash to buy food on her own, her taste buds went into overdrive and more and more she craved sugary and salty foods. I should have known something was up when the bag of baked chips I had purchased lasted longer than a week, and the trash can in her room started to look like she was taking daily trips to Willy Wonka's Chocolate Factory.

The more creative I got with meal preparation, the more she reached for the salt shaker, and this really bothered me because I didn't want her unhealthy eating habits to follow her into adulthood. Desperate times call for desperate measures, so I decided to hide the salt from her. That worked for about a minute! The next day I discovered salt packets in her backpack, which she had brought home from the school cafeteria! Ok, she wants to play? I can play; shoot, I invented the game! On to Plan B, the intellectual approach. She's a smart kid, maybe if I show her some research on how consuming too much salt can have adverse effects on the body, she'll listen to me and change her salty ways! Yeah, right! For those of you who have teenagers, you knew this wasn't going to work before you finished reading the sentence, didn't you? Next!

They say necessity is the mother of invention, and I need her to stop eating so much salt! Sometimes words are not enough, and you have to stop talking and take action, hence Plan C. On my next run to the grocery store, instead of buying regular table salt, I buy Lite Salt; it has 50% less sodium than regular salt, but still tastes like salt and cooks like salt. As soon as I got home I quickly emptied all the salt shakers and refilled them with Lite Salt. I was able to make the switch without her ever noticing, and do you know it only took three weeks for her taste buds to change?

We were eating lunch at a restaurant one day, three weeks after I had conducted my little experiment and she did her usual thing of salting the food before she tasted it, I watched, fearing I had failed again, already coming up with Plan D. But this time when she took a bite of her food her faced frowned up, and she quickly reached for her water. "What's wrong?" I asked, hoping my instincts were right. She answered with a disgusted look, "Restaurant food is so salty. These fries are killing me!" I smiled triumphantly and watched as she feverishly tried to brush the salt off her French fries. "Yeah," I thought to myself, "I still got it!"

How Savvy are you about Sodium?

Let's test your salt (sodium) IQ! The goal here is to become an 'A' student at living a healthier lifestyle, not test taking, so don't worry if you don't know all the answers, just take a guess. By the end of the quiz, you'll be at the head of the class! Circle your answer to the questions below. [2]

1. There is a direct relationship between sodium intake and high blood pressure. T or F
2. How much sodium does your body need daily? 1000mg 2300mg 200mg None of the above

3. Most of the salt people consume is added at the table. T or F
4. When reading food labels for sodium count, baking soda should be counted toward the total. T or F
5. Kosher salt and Sea salt are low sodium alternatives. T or F
6. A cup of canned tomato juice has more sodium than an ounce of potato chips. T or F
7. Some over the counter and prescription drugs contain lots of sodium. T or F

Answers:
1. True – Too much sodium causes your body to retain water which puts an extra burden on your heart and blood vessels. Reducing the amount of sodium in your diet may help you lower or keep you from having high blood pressure.
2. 200mg– Your body doesn't need much sodium for daily functions.
3. False – Most of the salt we consume comes from processed prepackaged food.
4. True- Always look for baking soda (sodium bicarbonate) when reading labels. 1 teaspoon of baking soda contains 1,000mg of sodium.
5. False – Kosher salt and Sea salt are chemically the same as table salt. 40% sodium.
6. True– depending on the brand, tomato juice has 340 – 1040mg of sodium per 8oz can. One ounce of potato chips has 120-180mg.
7. True – Be sure to read the labels or ask your pharmacist. Some brands come in a low sodium formula.

So how did you do? Were you surprised by the answers? And most importantly, did you learn something? Well, here's a little more knowledge for you. The average American gets 4,000 –

6,000 milligrams of sodium per day. That's more than double the American Heart Association's recommended limit of 1,500 milligrams (a little less than one teaspoon). The CDC reports that 75 percent of sodium in the average American diet comes from salt added to processed or restaurant foods. In other words, we often don't even know we're eating it. So, while cutting table salt is a start, it may only be putting a tiny dent in your sodium intake if you aren't careful about what you eat.

Shaking the Salt Habit

More than 40 percent of African Americans have high blood pressure (hypertension).[3] Not only is high blood pressure more severe in blacks than whites, but it also develops earlier in life. By keeping your blood pressure in the healthy range, you are:

- Reducing your risk of your vascular walls becoming overstretched and injured
- Reducing your risk of your heart having to pump harder to compensate for blockages
- Protecting your entire body so that your tissue receives regular supplies of blood that is rich in the oxygen it needs
- Reducing your risk of heart attack, stroke, kidney disease and coronary artery disease

Adopting a healthy lifestyle is critical for the prevention of high blood pressure and plays a vital role in managing it. Simply decreasing your intake of sodium can help lower your blood pressure or prevent you from developing high blood pressure in the first place. So what can you do right now?

Tips for Reducing Sodium in Your Diet[4]

- Buy fresh, plain frozen, or canned with "no salt added" vegetables

- When cooking, use fresh poultry, fish and lean meat instead of canned or processed types
- Use herbs, spices and salt-free seasoning blends in cooking and at the table
- Cook rice, pasta and hot cereals without salt. Cut back on instant or flavored rice, pasta and cereal mixes which usually have added salt.
- Choose low sodium frozen dinners, pizza, packaged mixes, canned soup or broths and salad dressings
- Rinse canned foods (vegetables, tuna) to remove some of the sodium
- Always buy low or reduced sodium versions of foods
- READ LABELS! You only have 1500mg of sodium allowed per day. So choose wisely, it adds up!

Today's Challenge

Today I challenge you to really look at the amount of sodium you're eating each day, especially if you have high blood pressure. Be conscious of the foods you eat and make a mental note every time you pick up the salt shaker. Does your food really need salt or are you doing it out of habit? Check the kitchen cabinets and freezer for foods that have a high sodium content and then start replacing them with low sodium alternatives. Replace regular table salt with lite salt and look for alternative ways of seasoning the foods you eat. It won't take long for your taste buds to change and body to notice and feel the difference.

Day 3 Affirmation

"Trust in the LORD with all your heart and lean not on your own understanding; in all your ways acknowledge Him, and He will make your paths straight."

Proverbs 3:5-6

WHAT DID YOU LEARN FROM TODAY'S READING AND WHAT DID YOU LEARN ABOUT YOURSELF?

_____
_____
_____
_____
_____
_____
_____
_____
_____
_____
_____
_____

HOW WILL YOU TAKE ONE STEP TOWARDS LIVING A HEALTHIER LIFESTYLE TODAY?

_____
_____
_____
_____
_____
_____
_____
_____
_____
_____
_____

LIST THREE THINGS (ANY THING) YOU'RE PROUD OF YOURSELF FOR TODAY AND EXPLAIN WHY:

_____
_____
_____
_____
_____
_____
_____
_____
_____
_____
_____
_____
_____
_____
_____
_____

SPEND FIVE MINUTES TODAY RECONNECTING YOUR SPIRIT TO GOD. WRITE IT, PRAY IT OR SHOW IT!

_____
_____
_____
_____
_____
_____
_____
_____
_____
_____
_____
_____
_____
_____
_____
_____

Day 4
You CAN Eat a Meal without Bread

Flour, butter, sugar, shortening, water, salt and yeast. How can ingredients so simple turn into something so delicious?! I can remember my grandmother making fresh dinner rolls on special occasions. She had this huge mixing bowl that she would dump all the ingredients into and mix them with her hands. I loved to help her knead the dough (in my too-big apron) as she stood close by, "Don't play with it too long, you don't want it to get tough," she would say. She would cover the bowl containing the dough with one of her striped kitchen towels and place it near the stove to rise. Sometimes the urge got the best of me, and I would sneak a peek under the towel when Grandma wasn't looking. When the time was right Grandma would take the warm dough and place it on the kitchen counter which she had lightly dusted with flour. After she had rolled out the dough it was my job to cut it into perfect circles. Together we would take the circles, dip them in butter, pull them gently and fold them in half before placing them into a glass baking dish. Parker House rolls were everyone's favorite, and we would make dozens of them! Fifteen minutes in the oven was all it took to create something so delicate and sweet, it melted in your mouth. Ahh, the smell of freshly baked bread! They caused many a fight among the kids if one of us thought the other had eaten more.

Bread was a staple in the Smith household. My Grandma was diligent about making sure there was some kind of bread to go with every meal. As far as I knew, it was a sin not to make cornbread every day. Get caught without bread on the table if you want to; people will think you've lost your mind! Greens and cornbread, spaghetti and cornbread and cornbread as a snack! I loved the way you could walk into her house any day of the week and smell the delicious aroma of freshly baked bread. Biscuits for breakfast, biscuits for dinner. I mean, how else were you going to sop up syrup or gravy? Yes, I said it! And if you have spent any time in the South you know what I'm talking about so don't get all bougie now!

There's no denying people love bread. We need bread as part of a healthy diet. So what's wrong with eating a little bread every now and then? The problem is not bread itself; the issue lies in the type of bread you're eating and how your body digests it that could make it a problem for your body type. Bread, rolls, buns, croissants, bagels, muffins, doughnuts, pizza dough, etc., all start with the same ingredient--flour. Flour is made when a grain, usually wheat, but sometimes oats, barley, spelt, or corn, is ground into a powder. If the wheat kernel's bran, or outer shell, and the germ, which is the kernel's center, are removed, the result is **white flour**. If the bran and germ are not removed, the result is **whole-wheat flour.** Let's compare whole-wheat bread vs. white bread.

Whole-wheat bread is much higher in fiber, vitamins B6 and E, magnesium, zinc, folic acid and chromium. The most important of these ingredients is fiber. Fiber has long been known to aid in digestive health and can help you lose or maintain weight because eating fiber-dense wheat bread helps you feel full. In a Harvard study of 75,000 nurses, those who ate at least three servings a day of whole grains (oatmeal, brown rice, quinoa), cut their heart attack risk by 35% and were less likely to get into weight or bowel trouble. By contrast, those who ate more processed foods such as white bread or white rice were more than twice as likely to develop diabetes.* Simply switching from white to whole-wheat bread can lower heart disease risk by 20 percent! And since the whole-wheat kernel is a complex carb,

24

most people find it doesn't affect their glycemic index (blood sugar levels).[5]

White bread is made from refined flour and when flour is refined it loses the most nutritious parts of the grain—the fiber, essential fatty acids, and most of the vitamins and minerals. In fact, about 30 nutrients are removed, but by law, only five must be added back (though others often are): iron, niacin, thiamin, riboflavin and folic acid. There's so little fiber left after processing that you'd have to eat eight pieces of white bread to get the fiber in just one piece of whole-wheat bread.[5]

I think the picture is clear! If you're going to eat bread (or pasta) in any form, it has to be whole-wheat. When purchasing bread make sure you read the label; if the first ingredient is not **whole grain** or **whole-wheat** you're basically buying white bread that has had enough brown flour or caramel coloring added to it to give it the appearance of whole-wheat bread. So enjoy your bread every now and then but eat it in a smarter, healthier way. And remember, you *can* eat a meal without bread. Your body will thank you for it!

*Len Marquart, professor of nutrition at the University of Minnesota and author of the first health claim for whole grains approved by the US Food and Drug Administration.

Today's Challenge

Today I challenge you to change your perception of bread and see it for what it really is -- a grain. Your body doesn't need bread to survive, it needs grains. Give up bread, just for today, then start adding more whole grains to your meal plans. Also, check the cabinets and see where you can replace refined breads, rice and pastas with whole grains. Check the labels on cereals too!

Day 4 Affirmation

"Commit to the LORD whatever you do, and your plans will succeed."

Proverbs 16:3

WHAT DID YOU LEARN FROM TODAY'S READING AND WHAT DID YOU LEARN ABOUT YOURSELF?

_____

_____

_____

_____

_____

_____

_____

_____

_____

_____

_____

_____

HOW WILL YOU TAKE ONE STEP TOWARDS LIVING A HEALTHIER LIFESTYLE TODAY?

_____

_____

_____

_____

_____

_____

_____

_____

_____

_____

_____

_____

LIST THREE THINGS (ANY THING)YOU'RE PROUD OF YOURSELF FOR TODAY AND EXPLAIN WHY:

_____
_____
_____
_____
_____
_____
_____
_____
_____
_____
_____
_____
_____
_____
_____

SPEND FIVE MINUTES TODAY RECONNECTING YOUR SPIRIT TO GOD. WRITE IT, PRAY IT OR SHOW IT!

_____
_____
_____
_____
_____
_____
_____
_____
_____
_____
_____
_____
_____
_____
_____
_____
_____

Day 5
Potatoes: How Do I Love Thee, Let Me Count the Ways

Dear Lord, please cover Grandma's ears as I tell yet another story about her with love in my heart. And the church said, Amen!

My Grandparents, Robert and Marguerite Smith, were married in 1937. She was a beautiful, scrawny little thing of 22, and he was a tall and handsome young man of 23. They literally had nothing but love for each other as they started their married life together in the tiny house located in the backyard of my Great-Grandmother's house on Cypress Street. The little house had only three rooms and was built for my Great-Great Grandmother years before when she moved to Pueblo, Colorado from Birmingham, Alabama. As kids, we would spend hours in it playing games, reading, and coloring; it was the perfect playhouse. As soon as you walked through the front door you were in the kitchen. There was a stove, sink, icebox and a coal stove for heat. Yellow curtains with pink flowers hung above the sink in the small window. The kitchen was too small for a table, so it was placed in a little dining area off to the left. The bedroom, big enough for a double bed and dresser was straight ahead. Indoor plumbing was a luxury the little house didn't have so my Grandparents used the outhouse further back in the yard.

As a newlywed Grandma had a lot to learn. She wasn't afraid of hard work. She had done that most of her life, but taking care of a husband and raising a family was something different. At the time, cooking was not her strong point. She knew the basics because she often cooked for her brothers and sisters, but her repertoire was lacking, so when she got married and had to cook for her new husband, she did the best she could. She woke up early every morning to make him breakfast and pack his lunch, and she had dinner on the table as soon as he came home from work without fail. She kept the tiny house spotless, and his clothes were always clean and pressed. Let me just add right here, I hate to iron now. Can you imagine doing it with an iron you had to heat up on the stove?! But I digress, back to the story.

One day, Grandpa comes home from work and Grandma is setting the table, just waiting for him to wash his hands and sit down so she can take up the food. She worked hard on this meal for her husband and was proud to serve him. She had prepared cornbread, baked ham and boiled potatoes. Basic, but satisfying. The next night when Grandpa sat down for dinner there was cornbread, fried chicken, mashed potatoes and gravy. The night after that, they had cornbread, meatloaf and mashed potatoes. Grandpa was starting to sense a theme, but he didn't say anything. Times were hard, potatoes were cheap, and he was thankful for all blessings. The weekend came, and for dinner they had (say it with me) cornbread, fried catfish and fried potatoes with onions. Now Grandpa was a patient man, slow to anger but quick to set things straight if need be. So it took awhile for him to decide he needed to say something to Grandma about her meal selections. The next week as he sits down for dinner and notices they are eating potatoes yet again, he finally speaks up, "Marge, don't you know how to cook any other vegetable besides potatoes?" he said. "Well I thought you liked potatoes," she replied. "I do but not every night!" Grandpa said, as gently as he could.

Ultimately, Grandma took cooking lessons from my Great-Grandma and learned how to cook *everything* Grandpa liked to eat. Some of the foods she learned to cook like chitlins, pig feet and brains, I wish she hadn't! Ewww! But I'll save that for another chapter. We can laugh at this story today, but I know some of you are just as passionate about potatoes as my grandmother was. How many days of the week do you have potatoes? Hash browns in the morning, French fries or chips at lunch, and a baked potato for dinner because "it's better for you." Remember when we talked about body types and how our bodies can change from one type to another? And remember how the round shaped endomorph was more susceptible to heart disease than the others? Well, before you turn into a potato-loving, round endomorph, let's talk about carbs!

Test time! Put check marks by the options which contain carbohydrates.

a) A sandwich made on white bread
b) Spinach salad with tomatoes, carrots and kidney beans
c) French fries
d) A sandwich made on whole grain bread

If you checked all the answers you are correct! All the foods above are carbohydrates, but answers B and D contain good carbohydrates (whole grains and vegetables). How do you determine the difference between good carbs and bad carbs? It's easy. Let's take a look.

Good Carbs vs. Bad Carbs

Carbohydrates are your body's primary energy source and they are a critical part of any healthy diet. Carbs should never be avoided, but it is important to understand that not all carbs are alike. Carbohydrates can be either simple (bad) or complex (good) based on their chemical makeup and what your body does with them. [6]

Complex carbohydrates are considered "good" because of the longer series of sugars that make them up and take the body more time to break down. They generally have a lower glycemic index, which means that you will get lower amounts of sugars released at a more consistent rate, instead of peaks and valleys, to keep you going throughout the day. Good carbs are plant foods that deliver fiber, vitamins, minerals along with carbohydrates such as whole grains, beans, vegetables, fruits, and low-fat or skim milk. Fruits and vegetables are actually simple carbohydrates, but the fiber in them changes the way that the body processes their sugars and slows down their digestion, making them act more like complex carbohydrates. [6]

Simple carbohydrates are considered "bad" and are composed of simple-to-digest, basic sugars with little real value for your body. The higher in sugar and lower in fiber, the worse the carbohydrate is for you. Bad carbs include: Soda, candy, sugar, white rice, white bread, white pasta, potatoes (which are technically a complex carb, but act more like simple carbs in the body), pastries and desserts. You can enjoy simple carbohydrates every now and then, but they shouldn't be your primary source of carbs. [6]

Carbs and the Glycemic Index

The *glycemic index* of a food basically tells you how quickly and how high your blood sugar will rise after eating the carbohydrate contained in that food, as compared to eating pure sugar. Lower glycemic index foods are healthier for your body, and you will tend to feel full longer after eating them. Most, but not all, complex carbs fall into the low glycemic index category.

It is easy to determine which of these foods are good carbs or bad carbs based on their **glycemic index**. Place a check mark by answers you think are bad carbs.[6]

a) White rice, 64

b) Brown rice, 44

c) White spaghetti, 55

d) Whole wheat spaghetti, 37

e) Corn flakes, 81

f) 100 percent bran (whole grain) cereal, 38

If you answered, A, C and E you're correct! The glycemic index is higher in these foods than the others.[7]

There's been a lot of hype about carbs in the media. Some people say you shouldn't eat them and some people say you should. Bottom line is, our bodies need carbohydrates, they're part of a balanced diet, but we have to be smart about the way we eat them. For example, choose sweet potato fries over regular French fries, and ask for brown rice the next time you order Chinese food. Choosing nutrient rich foods over nutrient deficient foods can make an impact on the quality of life we live each day. Start today by taking this small step on your journey to living a healthier lifestyle. I know you want to! But more importantly, I know you can!

Today's Challenge

Today I challenge you to be mindful of the amount and type of carbs you eat today. Are they good carbs or bad carbs? If you're diabetic, pay attention to spikes in your blood sugar and determine if eating carbs was the trigger. Make an effort today to stay away from the bad carbs and choose more good carbs. You'll be amazed at how your body responds!

Day 5 Affirmation

"Don't you know that you yourselves are God's temple and that God's Spirit lives in you?"

1 Corinthians 3:16

WHAT DID YOU LEARN FROM TODAY'S READING AND WHAT DID YOU LEARN ABOUT YOURSELF?

_____

_____

_____

_____

_____

_____

_____

_____

_____

_____

_____

_____

HOW WILL YOU TAKE ONE STEP TOWARDS LIVING A HEALTHIER LIFESTYLE TODAY?

_____

_____

_____

_____

_____

_____

_____

_____

_____

LIST THREE THINGS (ANY THING)YOU'RE PROUD OF
YOURSELF FOR TODAY AND EXPLAIN WHY:

_____

_____

_____

_____

_____

_____

_____

_____

_____

_____

_____

_____

_____

_____

_____

_____

_____

_____

_____

SPEND FIVE MINUTES TODAY RECONNECTING YOUR
SPIRIT TO GOD. WRITE IT, PRAY IT OR SHOW IT!

_____

_____

_____

_____

_____

_____

_____

_____

_____

_____

_____

_____

_____

Day 6
I Used to Run Every Day. Now My Knees Hurt So Bad I Can't

When I was in my early thirties, I looked good! No really, I looked good! You couldn't tell me anything. I wore a size 8-10, my legs were perfectly toned, my butt wasn't melting into my thighs, and my boobs looked up and out at the world as if to say, "Haaaaay!" I didn't have to exercise and I could eat anything and everything and not gain an ounce. One of my favorite memories of this blissful, pre-gravity time in my life is of pizza night with my daughter. As a single mother, you have to get creative with entertainment for your kids. Money is always tight. So, I came up with pizza night! Every Friday after work I would pick up my daughter from afterschool care at the Y, and we would drive to Blockbuster to grab some movies. Along the way, we would catch up on each other's day; she would tell me what happened at school and I would vent about the traffic, or my coworkers. We couldn't wait to get home, get comfortable and order pizza! We spent a lot of Friday nights in our pajamas watching movies on the floor, eating pizza right out of the box. Pure Heaven!

Then one day, I turned 38. I heard screeching sounds, looked out the window and saw my metabolism coming to an abrupt halt. Overnight (because eating a large pizza every Friday night had nothing to do with it) I had gained 40 pounds! Now, what I'm about to tell you has got to stay between you and me, because putting it in a book for the world to read would be too embarrassing, okay? I had just taken a shower, turned off the water and was about to reach for the towel, when I decided to shake off. You know, the way a dog does. So I did. Suddenly I stopped, frozen with fear; what was that noise? I listened and listened but heard nothing. "Oh great, now my mind is going too!" I thought as I proceeded to shake again. This time the sound was unmistakable; I looked down at my thighs, shook one more time and gasped as I realized that the sound was coming from ME! My thighs were slapping together! I had gotten so big, my thighs were slapping together! Mortified, I ran out of the shower and looked in the mirror. I couldn't believe what I saw! The woman who stared back at me from the glass had my face but was wearing someone else's body.

Do you remember the first time you looked in the mirror and saw someone else? How many pounds had you gained? I didn't know what to do; so I cried. I was scared. I had never dieted in my life! Unfortunately, the fear manifested itself as denial, and I kept right on eating. "I still look good," I tried to convince myself as I reached for the size 16 skirt on the rack. Two years passed and I was sitting on the table in my doctor's office complaining of knee pain. "I don't know what's wrong. Every time I climb a flight of stairs my knees hurt. I used to run every day but now even walking hurts," I told her. She ordered x-rays and gave me a complete physical. When I went back for the follow up visit, I just knew the test results were going to be bad. I was positive I had some mysterious disease no one could cure, but would make a great Lifetime movie after I was dead. I prayed as I sat in the car knowing that whatever it was I could handle it. God doesn't put more on us than we can bear, right?

My doctor explained that nothing negative had showed up in the test results, and I breathed a sigh of relief. Then she said the unthinkable, "Maybe if you lose a few pounds your knees will stop hurting." Excuse me?! Did she just say that to ME?! Note to self, find another doctor! There I sat in pain and she suggests

36

losing a few pounds?! Well here's a novel idea for you, how about writing me a prescription for the pain! I wobbled right out of that exam room, plopped my huge behind onto the seat of my car and drove away. Thank goodness it was Friday; at least I had pizza to look forward to!

It took a couple of months for me to open my eyes to the reality about my weight gain and decide to take action. My plan was to start walking and learn more about how to lose weight. This was around the time when that big media campaign about walking 10,000 steps was going on, so I bought a pedometer and started counting my steps. Every day after work I would walk. Sometimes my daughter would walk with me; it was great. She was my motivator, "Come on Mom, catch up to me!"she would say as she ran past me, and I would lumber after her, my aching 40 year old knees going as fast as they could.

I worked through the pain, and it wasn't long before I was up to 4 miles a day. I walked four, sometimes five days a week and my body morphed. The tone came back in my legs, my stomach went down, my arms firmed up, my behind found its rightful place again and guess what -- my knees stopped hurting! I was almost embarrassed to go back to the doctor for that year's physical exam; I mean, who wants to admit they were wrong. My doctor couldn't believe it when she read the chart and saw that I had lost 35 pounds. "What have you done with yourself?" she joked. I was proud to tell her I had started exercising and eating right, like it was my idea.

I tell you this story because I want you to know that we all go through it. As women, our bodies are in a constant state of flux. We go through changes that would bring a strong man to his knees! Periods, cramps, childbirth, cramps, pap smears, mammograms, migraines, more cramps and menopause. We don't know what size we'll be from one month to the next, much less year to year. But we don't have to lose control. Obesity is a killer and just like all chronic diseases, it sneaks up on you one calorie at a time. It wasn't hard for me to identify the cause of my 40 pound weight gain; I was eating more fat and calories than I could burn! Basically, I was eating to satisfy my mouth and not my body. How many of you eat when you're not even hungry? How many times have you gone back to the buffet for a second plate of food just because you could? When was the last time you ate because you were stressed, mad, sad, or happy? How many unexplained aches and pains are you suffering from? And how long are you going to live in denial before you start living a healthier lifestyle? Well, I'm here to tell you, you're better than that! And honestly, if I can do it, so can you. So what's holding you back? Take your next step today towards living a healthier lifestyle, and I'll be right here cheering you on!

Today's Challenge

Today I challenge you to think about the reasons why you overeat. It might be something that goes back to your childhood or it could be your way of dealing with stress. I challenge you to make a mental note every time you eat and decide right then and there, am I eating to satisfy my mouth, an emotion or my body? If you're not eating to satisfy your body, you're sabotaging the healthier lifestyle you're trying to achieve.

Day 6 Affirmation

"Obviously, I'm not trying to win the approval of people, but of God. If pleasing people were my goal, I would not be Christ's servant."
Galatians 1:10

WHAT DID YOU LEARN FROM TODAY'S READING AND WHAT DID YOU LEARN ABOUT YOURSELF?

_____
_____
_____
_____
_____
_____
_____
_____
_____
_____
_____
_____

HOW WILL YOU TAKE ONE STEP TOWARDS LIVING A HEALTHIER LIFESTYLE TODAY?

_____
_____
_____
_____
_____
_____
_____
_____
_____
_____

LIST THREE THINGS (ANY THING)YOU'RE PROUD OF
YOURSELF FOR TODAY AND EXPLAIN WHY:

_____
_____
_____
_____
_____
_____
_____
_____
_____
_____
_____
_____
_____
_____
_____
_____
_____
_____

SPEND FIVE MINUTES TODAY RECONNECTING YOUR
SPIRIT TO GOD. WRITE IT, PRAY IT OR SHOW IT!

_____
_____
_____
_____
_____
_____
_____
_____
_____
_____
_____
_____
_____

Day 7
Grandma Did It, Mama Did It, I'll Do It

H ave you ever heard the story about the pot roast? It's not my personal story, it came to me in one of those chain emails. You know, the ones that say, "Send this to 150 people including me in the next 5 seconds and God will bless you." Don't you hate those?! Am I the only one who wonders how God managed to answer all those prayers BEFORE the internet? The story is short, but the message it conveys is profound. So, if you have friends like mine and received this story in an email, I hope that after reading it in this context you'll see it in a whole new light. If this is your first time reading it, enjoy!

A young woman is preparing a pot roast while her friend looks on. She cuts off both ends of the roast, prepares it and puts it in the pan. "Why do you cut off the ends?" her friend asks. "I don't know," she replies. "My mother always did it that way and I learned how to cook it from her."

Her friend's question made her curious about her pot roast preparation. During her next visit home, she asked her mother, "How do you cook a pot roast?" Her mother proceeded to explain and added, "You cut off both ends, prepare it and put it in the pot and then in the oven." "Why do you cut off the ends?" the daughter asked. Baffled, the mother offered, "That's how my mother did it and I learned it from her!"

Her daughter's inquiry made the mother think more about the pot roast preparation. When she next visited her mother in the nursing home, she asked, "Mom, how do you cook a pot roast?" The mother slowly answered, thinking between sentences. "Well, you prepare it with spices, cut off both ends and put it in the pot." The mother asked, "But why do you cut off the ends?" The Grandmother's eyes sparkled as she remembered. "Well, the roasts were always bigger than the pot that we had back then. I had to cut off the ends to fit it into the pot that I owned."

Isn't that a great story?! I immediately took inventory of all the things I do just because my mother or grandmother did them, and it made me think about the traditions I'm handing down to my daughter. As African American's, we hold our family traditions close to our hearts; they've become the tapestry of our lives, each one woven with the blood, sweat and tears of the generations that came before us. They comfort us, make us feel loved and always bring us back together. The way we cook is one of those traditions (some people call it soul food) and just like the family in the story, we've handed down recipes from one generation to the next without ever stopping to ask, why?

My grandma cooked with things like, fat back, shortening, sugar, salt and *real* butter. She made meals from scratch, and there was nothing low fat or low calorie about them. In her house, butter was considered the fifth food group! But she cooked the way she did because, at the time, there were no healthier options. She used butter because there was no such thing as margarine. She used salt because Mrs. Dash didn't exist or shortening because Crisco hadn't figured out how to unsaturate oils yet. Now I will admit that there are some recipes I won't change, like the cookie recipe that calls for a pound of butter. We only make them once a year at Christmas so I'm going to enjoy! But there are others I wouldn't dream of making as is! Like her recipe for collard greens, I don't know what fat back is or where it comes from, and I most certainly don't want it in my collard greens!

It's vital for you to see the correlation between what we eat and the way it affects our bodies, so let's go back to the list of chronic diseases to see what causes them and then learn what we can do to prevent them.

Cardiovascular Disease	Smoking, <u>obesity</u>, <u>eating foods high in saturated fat</u>, stress, lack of exercise
High Blood Pressure	<u>Salt intake</u>, age, lack of exercise, <u>obesity</u>, stress, excessive alcohol consumption, sleep apnea, <u>family history</u>
High Cholesterol	<u>Obesity</u>, <u>eating foods high in saturated fat</u>, lack of exercise, <u>family history</u>
Obesity	<u>Unhealthy diet and eating habits</u>, lack of exercise, smoking, excessive alcohol consumption, <u>eating foods high in saturated fat, sugar, salt</u>, stress, lack of sleep, certain medications
Diabetes	Race, age, <u>obesity</u>, lack of exercise, high blood pressure, smoking, excessive alcohol consumption, <u>family history</u>

*American Heart Association Statistical Fact Sheet Update, 2012

With the chronic disease rate higher for us than any other race, our ignorance or complacency about food is literally killing us! Soul food is typically high in saturated fats, sodium, and sugar so the food we love is the very thing that is putting our lives at risk. Here are a couple of examples in case you have any doubts:

Based on one serving:

Chicken and Waffles

911 cal. 240 calories from fat (35% saturated fat)   775mg sodium

Chitlins

263 cal. 22,900mg of fat (10,800mg saturated fat)   20mg sodium

Now I know you don't eat chitlins every day; if you did you wouldn't be reading this book right now! But if you continue to eat foods that are high in fat, sodium and sugar you <u>will</u> gain weight and you <u>will</u> develop chronic disease. I'm sorry, but that's the truth! So what can you do right now to start towards your goal of healthy eating? Here are some simple changes you can make right now that will have an immediate impact on your health.

Fried Food Alternatives

Substitute lean, oven-baked chicken breast for deep-fried chicken, and baked sweet potato fries for deep-fried onion rings and French fries. Use roasting, sautéing or steaming methods to cook other meats and vegetables that are sometimes deep-fried, such as ham steaks and okra. Poached or grilled salmon provides the same amount of protein as deep-fried fish without all the saturated fat and cholesterol while adding heart-healthy omega-3 fish oils.[8]

Vegetable and Fruit Dishes

Keep the tradition of using plentiful, vitamin-rich vegetables in your menus, but use healthy flavoring agents and cooking methods. Cooked kale and collards, mustard, turnip or beet greens are packed with iron, calcium and vitamins A and C, among other nutrients. Casseroles or side dishes relying on sweet potatoes or yams are full of antioxidants, as are green beans and okra. Boost your daily vegetable servings by topping meats and side dishes with tomato sauce or salsa instead of fat-laden butter or gravy. Keep the tradition of fruit and vegetable-based desserts such as banana pudding, peach cobbler and sweet potato pie alive; simply adjust the recipes by using vegetable oil in place of shortening and butter, as well as incorporating fat-free versions of milk, evaporated milk, whipped cream and instant pudding.[9]

Cut Fat and Cholesterol

Use 1 percent buttermilk and vegetable oil in biscuits and cornbread. Make a healthier version of macaroni and cheese from low-fat cheddar, egg whites and evaporated fat-free milk or 2% milk. Replace bacon with turkey bacon and use nonfat vegetable cooking spray instead of butter or shortening to grease the casserole dishes.

Include Whole Grains

Use wheat and stone ground corn flour for cornbread instead of white and extra-refined corn meal to increase your intake of complex carbohydrates and dietary fiber. Season casseroles and breaded food with wholegrain bread crumbs or cereal flakes. Rice dishes such as red beans and rice or jambalaya are staples of some soul food recipes. Using brown rice instead of white rice makes these healthy meals even healthier by adding complex carbs. Add fiber to meatloaf by using oatmeal or wholegrain breadcrumbs in place of white bread crumbs or crackers.[10]

Healthier Seasoning Tips

Smoked turkey neck, herbs, spices and sea salt are useful alternatives to high-sodium, high-fat foods such as ham hocks and fat back. Smoked turkey necks in particular gives foods the "smokey" taste you love without all the fat.[11]

So my question to you is, just because our grandmothers and mothers did it, do we have to do it? Some traditions we as black women can't afford to carry on. I want you to take a look at some of the recipes handed down in your family and see where substitutions can be made. Get creative, have fun with it and who knows, maybe you'll start a new family tradition, one of good health! Someone once said, "When you know better, you do better." So what are you waiting for? Do better!

Today's Challenge

Today I challenge you to look at the traditions your family has handed down as far as food is concerned. How have they influenced the way you think about food? Are they impacting your health in a negative way? If so, give yourself permission to make changes where necessary for the sake of your health. Grandma will still be proud!

Day 7 Affirmation

"Know therefore that the LORD your God is God, the faithful God who keeps covenant and steadfast love with those who love him and keep his commandments, to a thousand generations".

Deuteronomy 7:9

WHAT DID YOU LEARN FROM TODAY'S READING AND WHAT DID YOU LEARN ABOUT YOURSELF?

_____
_____
_____
_____
_____
_____
_____
_____
_____
_____
_____
_____

HOW WILL YOU TAKE ONE STEP TOWARDS LIVING A HEALTHIER LIFESTYLE TODAY?

_____
_____
_____
_____
_____
_____
_____
_____
_____
_____

LIST THREE THINGS (ANY THING)YOU'RE PROUD OF
YOURSELF FOR TODAY AND EXPLAIN WHY:

_____
_____
_____
_____
_____
_____
_____
_____
_____
_____
_____
_____
_____
_____
_____
_____
_____
_____

SPEND FIVE MINUTES TODAY RECONNECTING YOUR
SPIRIT TO GOD. WRITE IT, PRAY IT OR SHOW IT!

_____
_____
_____
_____
_____
_____
_____
_____
_____
_____
_____
_____
_____
_____

Day 8
Red, Purple, and Orange are Colors, NOT DRINKS

R ed, purple, yellow, orange, green, and pink; I had no clue how to spell Lemon-Lime and I didn't care, all I knew was that green Kool-Aid was my favorite! Ask any black family with or without kids under the age of 25 if they have Kool-Aid readily made, chilling in the fridge and the answer will be YES! Kool-Aid is cheap, and it does the job. It quenches your thirst, gives you energy (in a bouncing off the walls sort of way), and it has Vitamin C! I still keep four or five colorful packets in my kitchen even though my child is out of the house and I don't drink it anymore. It's kind of comforting I guess. It makes me feel like a real Mom if I can produce a pitcher of Kool-Aid for a bunch of thirsty kids. I get all sentimental when I walk down the aisle of the grocery store and see Kool-Aid's smiling face looking back at me from the shelf. The commercial plays in my head and on cue I shout, "Hey, Kool-Aid!" Yes, those were the days! As a kid, I didn't have to worry about what I ate OR drank, in fact, the more sugar the better! Pixie Stix, Dots, candy necklaces, Reese's and my all time favorite: Hot Tamales! Ice cream sandwiches, soda pop, candy apples, and popsicles. Whew! I get a sugar rush just thinking about it! It was a simpler time back then, the days when red, purple and green were more than just colors, they were the names of our favorite drinks.

How Much Sugar Do We Eat?

The United States Department of Agriculture (USDA) reports that the **average American consumes anywhere between 150 to 170 pounds of simple sugars, also known as refined sugars (this includes glucose, fructose, and sucrose) or simple carbohydrates, in one year!** Less than 100 years ago, the average intake of sugar was *only* about 4 pounds per person per year.

Can't get a grasp on how much sugar 150 to 170 pounds is? Here is a visual: imagine 30 to 34 five-pound bags of sugar lined up next to each other on a counter. Now imagine one person, perhaps yourself, eating all of that sugar. To break it down even more, eating 150-170 pounds of sugar in one year is also equivalent to consuming 1/4 to 1/2 pounds of sugar *each day,* that's 720 extra calories for each day of the week! If you're still not convinced, I'll break it down even further:

There are 120 teaspoons in one pound of sugar. This means 1/4 pound of sugar is equivalent to 30 teaspoons, and 1/2 pound of sugar is equivalent to 60 teaspoons. An average 12-ounce can of soda contains about 8 ounces of simple sugar. This means that just four 12-ounce cans of sodas (48 ounces) will equal 1/4 pound of sugar! For some people, drinking this amount of soda, sweet tea or Kool-Aid in one day is not a difficult task to accomplish.

Now think about the *other* sources of sugar in our diet like; doughnuts, candy, cookies, cake, and ice cream. Or foods that contain sweeteners such as high fructose corn syrup like salad dressings, breads, hot dogs, peanut butter, pickles, canned fruits and vegetables, ketchup, canned soups, crackers, fruit drinks, fruit punch and ades.[12]

Packaged food

Refined sugar is hidden in a number of ways on the labels of packaged foods. Most ingredients that end in "ose" are a form of refined sugar. Other names that indicate refined sugar is added to packaged food include corn syrup, hydrolyzed starch, high fructose corn syrup, molasses, cane sugar, corn sweetener, raw sugar, syrup, honey, fruit juice concentrates and maltose. The total amount of sugar in a packaged food is listed under the carbohydrate column on labels. Nutritionists at the Food Standards Agency report that packaged food with **fewer than 5g of carbohydrates are low in refined sugars**, while foods that are listed as having more than 15g per serving are loaded. There are four calories in each gram, so if a product has 15 grams of sugar per serving, that's 60 calories just from the sugar alone, not counting the other ingredients. Food labels list ingredients in order of quantity, with the highest amounts listed first. Foods low in refined sugar list any sugars as the last ingredients.[13]

How Does it Affect Your Body?

Your body turns sugar into triglycerides, a type of fat that acts like LDL or "bad" cholesterol in your bloodstream. Eating too much refined sugar adds extra calories to your diet and if you consume more calories than you burn daily, you will gain weight, especially in the stomach area. **Adding just 100 calories extra of refined sugars daily will result in over 10 extra pounds gained over the course of a year!** All types of sugar can lead to weight gain, and we know that obesity leads to the development of clogged arteries, chronic conditions such as Type 2 diabetes, some cancers and heart disease.

Natural Sweeteners

Stevia, which is an herb, and xylitol, which is made from fruit and vegetable fibers are two forms of natural sugar that can add sweetness to a product without the harmful side effects associated with refined sugar. Agave nectar and honey are natural sugar foods that also provide a good source of carbohydrates needed for energy. Agave nectar is 90% fructose which can be a concern, but because of its low glycemic index it doesn't spike your blood sugar levels like processed sugar.[14]

Artificial Sweeteners

Artificial sweeteners are synthetic sugar substitutes but may be derived from naturally occurring substances, including herbs or sugar itself. Artificial sweeteners are also known as intense sweeteners because they are many times sweeter than regular sugar. Examples include:

- Sucralose – Splenda (Made from sugar)
- Truvia – (Made from herbs)
- Aspartame - Equal, NutraSweet (Synthetic)
- Saccharin - SugarTwin, Sweet'N Low (Synthetic) [15]

Artificial sweeteners are attractive alternatives to sugar because they add virtually no calories to your diet; however, research has also shown that regular use of artificial sweeteners may actually cause you to *gain* weight. Use them in moderation and be aware of potential side effects that could affect your health. For example, aspartame has been shown to increase respiratory problems, especially in people with asthma.

Tips for Reducing Sugar in Your Diet

The American Heart Association says most American women should limit their intake of **added sugars** to no more than 100 calories per day or about 6 tsp. of sugar*. So, if you've already had a can of soda today, you're done! But don't beat yourself up about it! The craving for sugar is a hard habit to break, so unless you're really disciplined, don't try to quit cold turkey, reduce the amount you eat gradually. Instead of drinking soda five times a week for lunch, switch to water one day a week, then two days a week and so on until you've given up soda completely. Below are more tips to reducing sugar in your diet.

*Amounts will vary based on your health and activity level. Check with your doctor to determine what's right for you.

- Don't buy it! Buy sugar only when needed for baking and then buy only what you need
- Drink water at meal time
- Dilute juices. Pour half a glass (or less) of juice then fill it up with water
- Avoid the vending machine, take healthy snacks to work with you
- At restaurants, order unsweetened tea and sweeten it yourself preferably with an artificial sweetener!
- Read the label! If it has more than 6 grams of sugar per serving, don't buy it!
- Buy sugar-free or low-calorie beverages
- Buy fresh fruits or fruits canned in water or natural juice. Avoid fruit canned in syrup, especially heavy syrup
- Instead of adding sugar to cereal or oatmeal, add fresh fruit (try bananas, cherries or strawberries) or dried fruit (raisins, cranberries or apricots) and use soy milk instead of regular milk
- When baking cookies, brownies or cakes, cut the sugar called for in your recipe by one-third. You won't notice the difference!
- Substitute unsweetened applesauce for sugar in recipes (use equal amounts)
- Stop the craving **before** it starts! Do not skip meals. This can lower your blood sugar levels, which cause you to crave that sugar for a quick fix. Eat protein rich, fiber filled foods to ward off hunger.[16]

Sugar and Your Hormones

As women, it's not easy for us to kick the sugar habit because of the sugar monster that visits us on a monthly basis. He casts a spell over us and makes us believe there's nothing wrong with eating half a dozen doughnuts in the car on the way home from work. Not that I've done that before, I'm just sayin'! The best advice I can give for these times is to get in tune with your body. Before you lay out the blanket and have a dessert orgy in the middle of the living room floor, stop and think about what's happening. Are you feeding your body or your mouth? Are you honestly hungry or just feeding hormones? Once you realize you're just feeding your hormones you can put the whipped cream down and choose a healthy sweet treat instead, like fruit!

Today's Challenge

Today I challenge you to identify ways you can reduce the amount of sugar in your diet. Read the labels on the food in your cabinets and look for reduced or sugar free alternatives. And try exercising through your cravings. When the urge for something sweet hits, take your mind off it by exercising for ten minutes, your body will thank you for it!

Day 8 Affirmation

"Now faith is the substance of things hoped for, the evidence of things not seen."

Hebrews 11:1

WHAT DID YOU LEARN FROM TODAY'S READING AND WHAT DID YOU LEARN ABOUT YOURSELF?

_____

_____

_____

_____

_____

_____

_____

_____

_____

_____

_____

_____

HOW WILL YOU TAKE ONE STEP TOWARDS LIVING A HEALTHIER LIFESTYLE TODAY?

_____

_____

_____

_____

_____

_____

_____

_____

_____

_____

_____

LIST THREE THINGS (ANY THING)YOU'RE PROUD OF
YOURSELF FOR TODAY AND EXPLAIN WHY:

_____

_____

_____

_____

_____

_____

_____

_____

_____

_____

_____

_____

_____

_____

_____

_____

SPEND FIVE MINUTES TODAY RECONNECTING YOUR
SPIRIT TO GOD. WRITE IT, PRAY IT OR SHOW IT!

_____

_____

_____

_____

_____

_____

_____

_____

_____

_____

_____

_____

_____

_____

Day 9
Fried Food Says, "I Love You"

Correct me if I'm wrong, but nothing says summer cook-out like deep fried cat fish. Tell me if I'm lying when I say Sunday dinner isn't complete without fried chicken and fried okra. Slap my face if you wouldn't rather have fried turkey over baked on Thanksgiving Day. And don't tell me you've never eaten a fried bologna sandwich. If you haven't, you're not black! Fried shrimp, fried potatoes and onions, fried eggs, fried green tomatoes; black folks will drop almost anything into a pan of hot grease and call it lunch. And why not, fried food tastes good! There's nothing more tantalizing than biting into a piece of crispy fried chicken; the crunch of the delicate skin as it breaks apart between your teeth releasing the explosion of warm juices onto your tongue, tormenting your taste buds with savory spices until your mouth is begging, yearning for you to bite deeper, deeper into the moist, tender meat. Your senses coming alive with every bite until finally, your body convulses with excitement and your mouth cries out for more, more, more! Did it just get hot in here, or is it me? Uh um, as I was saying, to put a twist on an old saying, "Everything that *tastes* good to you, ain't good for you!" The love triangle between black women, fried food and their bodies has been a tumultuous affair. It has turned us into crazed lunatics, driving all over town looking for the one thing that we know can satisfy us like no other, Mr. Bojangles or his older brother KFC. Our eyes light up at the sight of him and goose bumps form as we sit in anticipation at the drive thru. Our bodies aching, longing to hear those three little words, "Order when ready!" Believe me when I say I wish I could wave a magic wand and make fried food have the same caloric content and health benefits as vegetables, but I can't, so before we get all hot and bothered again by fantasizing about eating funnel cakes and fried ice cream, let's remember why we're here and take today to learn about fats. It's time to kick the fat to the curb. Are you with me? Let's do this!

The Truth About Fats and Frying

The fact is we all need fats. Fats help with nutrient absorption, nerve transmission, maintaining cell membrane integrity, etc. However, when consumed in excess amounts, fats contribute to weight gain, heart disease and certain types of cancer. But all fats are not created equal. Some fats promote our health positively while others increase our risks of heart disease. The key is to replace bad fats with good fats in our diet.

Frying foods increases the fat content and calories of the meal. Different types of frying include sautéing, stir frying, pan frying and deep frying. Sautéing and stir-frying add the least amount of calories; however, pan and deep frying can add many calories, especially when foods are coated with batter before frying (chicken, fish, pork chops). It's important for you to know the types of fats and how they differ so you can make healthier choices when preparing meals. Let's take a look. There are four types of fats used to fry foods; saturated fats, trans fats, monounsaturated fats and polyunsaturated fats.

Saturated Fat

Saturated fats remain solid at room temperature, and most are found in animal fat; although tropical plant oils are high in saturated fat. Lard, butter, and shortening are the most common saturated fats used in frying. **Overconsumption of saturated fat is associated with a higher risk of cardiovascular disease.** Adding this type of fat to your daily diet is not necessary; your body makes some saturated fat naturally, so it's something you don't need to eat to survive.

Trans Fat

Trans fats are semi-solid at room temperature, so they are useful for making stick margarine and shortenings. The trans fats used in cooking are artificially created when hydrogen atoms are forced into vegetable oils by a process called hydrogenation. Partially hydrogenated fats are more stable than regular vegetable oil, so they can be stored longer without going bad. **When you eat trans fats you increase your risk for cardiovascular disease.**

Monounsaturated Fat

Monounsaturated fats are liquid at room temperature but solid at cold temperatures. Olive oil is the monounsaturated fat most commonly used for stir-frying and sautéing. Canola and peanut oils contain monounsaturated fats, along with polyunsaturated fats. **Monounsaturated fats have positive health effects; research shows they can improve cholesterol levels and reduce inflammation in the body.**

Polyunsaturated Fat

Polyunsaturated fats are liquid at room temperature and at cool temperatures. Vegetable oils such as canola, soybean, corn, sunflower and safflower oils are mostly polyunsaturated fats. Consumption of polyunsaturated fats is associated with decreased risk of cardiovascular disease, especially a type of polyunsaturated fat called omega-3 fats. **Your body cannot make omega-3 fats, so they need to be part of your diet.** [17]

Knowing the Difference Between Healthy Fats and Harmful Fats

Below are the best food sources of these **healthy fats:** [18]

Type of healthy fat	Food source
Monounsaturated fat	Olive oil, peanut oil, canola oil, avocados, nuts and seeds

| Polyunsaturated fat | Vegetable oils (such as safflower, corn, sunflower, soy and cottonseed oils), nuts and seeds |
| Omega-3 fatty acids | Fatty, cold-water fish (such as salmon, mackerel and herring), flaxseeds, flax oil and walnuts |

Harmful fats

Saturated and trans fats (trans-fatty acids) are less healthy kinds of fats. They can increase your risk of heart disease by increasing your total and LDL ("bad") cholesterol. Dietary cholesterol isn't technically a fat, but it's found in food derived from animal sources. Intake of dietary cholesterol increases blood cholesterol levels, but not as much as saturated and trans fats do, and not to the same degree in all people.

Below are common food sources of harmful fats: [18]

Type of harmful fat	Food source
Saturated fat	Animal products (such as meat, poultry, seafood, eggs, dairy products, lard and butter), and coconut*, palm and other tropical oils *Although coconut oil is high in saturated fat, research shows the health benefits of using this oil make it a viable healthy alternative.
Trans fat	Partially hydrogenated vegetable oils, commercial baked goods (such as crackers, cookies and cakes), fried foods (such as doughnuts and French fries), shortening and margarine
Dietary cholesterol	Animal products (such as meat, poultry, seafood, eggs, dairy products, lard and butter)

Fast food restaurants and other eateries often use trans fats for frying foods. Trans fats can clog your arteries and increase your risk of cardiovascular disease, including coronary heart disease, heart attack and death. Research shows that trans fats can deplete your levels of HDL cholesterol, the good cholesterol that your body needs.

Tips For Choosing the Best Types of Fat

Limit fat in your diet, but don't try to cut it out completely. Focus on reducing foods high in saturated fat, trans fat and cholesterol, and select more foods made with unsaturated fats. Consider these tips when making your choices:

- Sauté with olive oil instead of butter.
- Use olive oil in salad dressings and marinades. Use canola oil when baking.
- Sprinkle slivered nuts or sunflower seeds on salads instead of bacon bits.
- Snack on a small handful of nuts rather than potato chips or processed crackers. Or try peanut butter or other nut-butter spreads (nonhydrogenated) on celery, bananas, or rice or popcorn cakes.
- Add slices of avocado, rather than cheese, to your sandwich.
- Prepare fish such as salmon and mackerel, which contain monounsaturated and omega-3 fats, instead of meat one or two times a week.[19]

Monounsaturated and polyunsaturated fats have few adverse effects on blood cholesterol levels, but you still need to consume all fats in moderation. Eating large amounts of any fat adds excess calories. Also, make sure that fatty foods don't replace more nutritious options, such as fruits, vegetables, beans or whole grains.

You're at greater risk for high blood **cholesterol** and **heart disease** if you eat a diet that often includes deep-fried or breaded foods, which are high in fat. Diets high in **saturated fat** and cholesterol tend to raise total cholesterol and **LDL** (or bad) cholesterol. Foods that are fried or breaded tend to be very high in fat because they are cooked in fat. Ever notice when you bake chicken or turkey how the "drippings" collect in the pan? That's the fat draining from the meat. When you fry foods, such as chicken that already contain saturated fat, you're simply adding more fat to them!

How to Reduce Your Risk

Take these actions to have a healthier heart.

- If you don't know your blood cholesterol level, have it tested.
- Each day eat no more than 6 to 8 teaspoons of fats and vegetable oils. Remember to count those used in cooking. Choose fats and oils that are mostly unsaturated such as olive oil. Avoid or limit those that are highly saturated, such as lard or butter.
- Opt for cooking methods that use little or no fat. Rather than deep-fry or pan-fry, cook your food by steaming, baking, broiling, roasting, grilling, or stir-frying.
- Eat at least two servings of fish per week, cooked using one of these healthier methods, to help improve your cholesterol levels and the health of your heart.
- Limit your total fat intake to no more than 25 percent to 35 percent of your total daily calories.
- Limit your saturated fat intake to less than 7 percent of your total daily calories.
- Limit your cholesterol intake to less than 200 mg per day.[20]

There is a lesson on how to read labels on Day 19, it will help you figure out these percentages.

It's simple ladies; you are what you eat, so you can't expect to lose weight and reverse the effects of chronic disease if you're still eating a sausage or chicken biscuit for breakfast, hamburgers and French fries for lunch and the number two shrimp basket with fries and hushpuppies for dinner. Eating foods fried in unhealthy fats is the quickest way to gain 50 pounds and develop chronic disease. I know you love fried foods, trust me, I was right there with you until I decided I loved me more. How much do you love yourself? It must be a lot because you're reading this book. Let today be the day you open your mind to the possibilities of living a healthier lifestyle and know that you're not taking this journey alone; I'm with you every step of the way!

Today's Challenge

Today I challenge you to give up fried meats in favor of grilled or baked meats. Be conscious of the trans fats you're eating every time you grab a cookie, cupcake, or doughnut and switch to 2 percent or 1 percent milk. Today I challenge you to cut the bad fats out of your diet and out of your life!

Day 9 Affirmation

"Let us not lose our zeal in doing good, for in due season we will reap a reward, if we do not give up."

Galatians 6:9

WHAT DID YOU LEARN FROM TODAY'S READING AND WHAT DID YOU LEARN ABOUT YOURSELF?

_____

_____

_____

_____

_____

_____

_____

_____

_____

_____

_____

_____

HOW WILL YOU TAKE ONE STEP TOWARDS LIVING A HEALTHIER LIFESTYLE TODAY?

_____

_____

_____

_____

_____

_____

_____

_____

_____

_____

LIST THREE THINGS (ANY THING) YOU'RE PROUD OF YOURSELF FOR TODAY AND EXPLAIN WHY:

_____

_____

_____

_____

_____

_____

_____

_____

_____

_____

_____

_____

_____

_____

_____

SPEND FIVE MINUTES TODAY RECONNECTING YOUR SPIRIT TO GOD. WRITE IT, PRAY IT OR SHOW IT!

_____

_____

_____

_____

_____

_____

_____

_____

_____

_____

_____

_____

_____

Day 10
A Mixing Bowl Does Not a Serving Size Make

Remember when you were a kid and would wake up before the crack of dawn on Saturday mornings just to watch cartoons? Unlike other days of the week, no alarm clock was necessary; you literally sprang out of bed and raced to the TV so you wouldn't miss a second of your favorite show. Sometimes my brothers and I woke up at the same time and the stampede down the hall towards the living room looked like an episode of Roller Derby as we pushed and shoved each other out of the way. I may have been the only girl, but I was quick to trip a brother if need be! You see, back in the day there was only one TV for the household, so whoever got there first controlled the channel. Unscathed, we would sit on the couch or lie on the floor in our footy pajamas, mesmerized by the black and white images on the screen and laugh till our sides hurt!

Mom and Dad wouldn't get up until later so this was the one day of the week we were allowed to fix our own breakfast. I was the third sibling which meant I had very little rank. My two older brothers, who for some reason thought they were "in charge" of me and my younger brother, often turned something as simple as the making of a bowl of cereal into the Hunger Games. My oldest brother (Generalissimo) was in charge of getting the bowls out of the cabinet, and the second oldest (El Capitán) was responsible for divvying up the cereal rations to us Privates. As if in rank order, Generalissimo placed the bowls on the table in a straight line; two serving bowls, one regular bowl and a Sesame Street bowl, for the newest recruit. "Wait a minute! Your bowls are bigger than mine!" I protested. "That's because we're bigger than you," the General would say. "They all hold the same amount anyway," El Capitán was quick to add. Now, my mama didn't raise no fools, but I was out numbered so, what's a girl to do? She cries at the top of her lungs, that's what she does! Nothing moves quicker than a brother in fear of getting his behind whooped! The last thing you wanted to hear on a Saturday morning was Dad's footsteps coming down the hall to see what happened. And since I was Daddy's only princess my wails would not go unpunished. See, God has a way leveling the playing field!

For years I had to listen to the "Because I'm bigger" speech. I couldn't wait until I was big enough to do, eat, or watch whatever I wanted. "When I get big I'm gonna have my own house with my own TV and you guys can't come over!" I would shout as I ran to my room and closed the door. It wasn't until I actually did have my own place that I realized how certain memories tuck themselves away, deep in the recesses of your mind and don't come out until one day you're sitting on the couch, in your pajamas, with a mixing bowl full of cereal. "What are you doing?" the voice inside my head said. "Eating cereal, what does it look like?" I replied out loud. "Are you *trying* to look like a sumo wrestler?" the voice chided me. I pulled up my big girl panties and said, "Look, I've waited a long time to do whatever I want and nobody's going to stop me!" "You know you'll never fit into that dress Saturday night if you keep eating like this," the voice reminded me. I jumped up from the couch, ran to the sink and poured the whole bowl down the drain! So much for being big.

How Big is a Serving Size

Most of us think a serving size is however much we put on our plates! That wouldn't be so bad if the size of plates hadn't increased over the years. The amount of food you put on your plate is by definition a "portion." Your plate may hold two thighs and a breast, but the "serving size" for chicken is one chicken breast. Any more than that and you've eaten two servings or more! According to the National Heart, Lung and Blood Institute (NHLBI), a "serving" is a unit of measure used to describe the amount of food recommended from each of the four food groups. For instance: one slice of bread, one chicken breast, a half cup of cooked vegetables and one medium apple.

The easiest way to determine if you are eating the correct serving size is to read the Nutrition Facts on the label. Take Honey Nut Cheerios for example. According to the label a serving size is three-fourths cup. I'm willing to wager that's a lot less than what you're putting in your cereal bowl; am I right?

Every day, your body uses calories to perform activities such as breathing, digestion and moving around. If you eat more calories than needed for these activities, the extra calories are stored as fat. For an average adult, this means that eating 100 more calories a day causes a weight gain of about 1 pound in a month. And don't forget serving size when it comes to liquids! Thirty-two ounces of sweet tea for $1.00 may sound like a good deal but not to your waistline. No wonder we can't fit into the clothes we bought last summer![21]

Here are some tips to developing and maintaining proper portion control:

At Home:
- Use smaller dishes at mealtime.
- Serve food in the appropriate portion amounts and don't go back for seconds.
- Put away any leftovers in separate, portion-controlled amounts. Consider freezing the portions you likely won't eat for a while.
- Never eat out of the bag or carton.

- Don't keep platters of food on the table; you are more likely to "pick" at it or have a second serving without even realizing it.[21]

At Restaurants:

The average restaurant entree has about twice the number of calories most adults need in one meal.

- Ask for half or smaller portions.
- Eyeball your appropriate portion, set the rest aside and ask for a doggie bag right away. Servings at many restaurants are often big enough to provide meals for two days.
- If you have dessert, share.

At the Grocery Store:

- Beware of "mini-snacks" -- tiny crackers, cookies, and pretzels. Most people end up eating more than they realize, and the calories add up.
- Choose foods packaged in individual serving sizes and eat only one pack.
- If you're the type who eats ice cream out of the carton, pick up ice cream sandwiches or other individual size servings.

Maintaining or losing weight is a challenge and although standard serving sizes can seem small, the average American underestimates how many calories they are ingesting each day by 25 percent! So remember, your goal to a healthier lifestyle is a marathon, not a sprint. You didn't gain the weight overnight, and you won't lose it overnight either. Take your time, let your body adjust to all the new things you're teaching it and be proud of the small accomplishments you're making each day! I am!

Today's Challenge

Today I challenge you to become a conscious eater, fully aware of what you're eating, how it tastes and grateful for the meal before you. Watch portion sizes and remember, you're eating to satisfy and nourish your body, not your mouth.

Day 10 Affirmation

"LORD, you have assigned me my portion and my cup; you have made my lot secure. The boundary lines have fallen for me in pleasant places; surely I have a delightful inheritance. I will praise the LORD, who counsels me; even at night my heart instructs me. I have set the LORD always before me. Because he is at my right hand, I will not be shaken."

Psalm 16:5-8

WHAT DID YOU LEARN FROM TODAY'S READING AND WHAT DID YOU LEARN ABOUT YOURSELF?

_____

_____

_____

_____

_____

_____

_____

_____

_____

_____

_____

HOW WILL YOU TAKE ONE STEP TOWARDS LIVING A HEALTHIER LIFESTYLE TODAY?

_____

_____

_____

_____

_____

_____

_____

_____

_____

LIST THREE THINGS (ANY THING)YOU'RE PROUD OF
YOURSELF FOR TODAY AND EXPLAIN WHY:

_____
_____
_____
_____
_____
_____
_____
_____
_____
_____
_____
_____
_____
_____
_____
_____
_____
_____

SPEND FIVE MINUTES TODAY RECONNECTING YOUR
SPIRIT TO GOD. WRITE IT, PRAY IT OR SHOW IT!

_____
_____
_____
_____
_____
_____
_____
_____
_____
_____
_____
_____
_____
_____

Day 11
I Can Eat All I Want Before 8PM

When I make up my mind about something, you can consider it done! I'm researching online and reading books, buying videos and CD's, whatever it takes to accomplish the task. So when I decided to quit living in denial and live a healthier lifestyle, I did my research. Now granted, I fell for, and tried some of those lose weight quick schemes, but I chalk it up to experience and learned from my mistakes. One of those life lessons happened the day I was watching an infomercial about the latest diet book. The well-suited man spoke very convincingly about why his book was the greatest thing since sliced bread. Just watching him dialog with the show's host was enough to make you run to your purse and pull out your credit card. I sat there for a good 15 minutes writing down little tidbits of information when finally he said the magic words, "If you want to lose weight you have to stop eating after 8pm. If you're not hungry in the morning, you're eating too much food late at night." The words hit me like a lightning bolt and instantly I knew I had just found my new diet plan! "Wow, how easy is that!" I thought to myself. "Why didn't I think of that before? I can eat anything I want; I just have to do it before eight o'clock!" At least that's what I heard.

The next day I was on a mission, I got up early because I knew I had to eat breakfast before I went to work, I didn't want to miss any opportunity to eat! I took snacks to work, ate both before eleven o'clock. Went out to lunch with my coworkers, ate some cookies out of the vending machine for my afternoon snack and then headed home for dinner. I think it was about 6:30 the first time I went back to the kitchen to look for something else to eat, and 7:45 when I found myself standing in front of the fridge trying to decide if I had enough time to polish off the spaghetti and the ice cream, or just the ice cream.

When I look back now and think about how gullible I was to even think that would work, I kind of get mad! First at the guy selling misinformation and then at myself for believing it! Take a guess at how many pounds I lost by not eating after eight o'clock. What was that? Did you say zero? Yep! Now guess how many pounds I gained! Never mind, I'd rather not be reminded.

Time of Day and Weight Gain

Before I started my eating frenzy, which is exactly what it was, I was on a steady decline with my weight, I was eating healthier, taking my snacks to work and slowly but surely I was beginning to see a change in my body. After listening to the "weight loss guru" on TV, I started to gain back the weight I had worked so hard to lose. Why? Because even though I wasn't eating at night anymore, I was consuming more calories during the day than I had previously.

Recent studies revealed that when people ate three meals a day only 13 percent binged at night. When people skipped breakfast, 24 percent binged and when people skipped breakfast and lunch, 60 percent binged. When you spread your meals throughout the day you have better control of your eating habits. You feel less hungry and are less likely to overeat. So by eating breakfast, lunch, and dinner and planning snacks in between, you can help yourself lose weight as well as maintain better control of your eating throughout the day and night. And remember what we learned about metabolic rate and calories? A calorie is a calorie no matter what time of the day or night it is consumed. The only way to lose weight is to burn more calories than you eat, so eating late at night has little impact on your weight gain or loss.[22]

Losing Weight While Snacking Late

Not eating after a certain time does not help you lose weight, but following set guidelines about your nighttime eating habits can. Eat at night only when you feel hungry, not just because you're bored, and eat low-calorie, nutritious foods in controlled portions while minimizing distractions. Skip the candy and opt for choices like string cheese, low-fat yogurt or apple slices spread with natural peanut butter.

So, let's make a new Snack Attack Plan, shall we? To do this, we don't necessarily need to trade all of our Chips Ahoy cookies in for carrot sticks or our carton of ice cream for a carton of yogurt. We can start by making smarter snack choices *most* of the time. Here are 10 tips on how you can do this each day:

Tip 1: Eat Snacks Loaded with Fiber

Foods rich in soluble fiber make for great snacks because soluble fiber leaves the stomach slowly, encouraging better blood sugars and making you feel satisfied longer. See the Fiber Rich Foods List on Day 20.

Tip 2: Eat Slow-Release Snack Foods

The following foods even in large amounts and if eaten alone, are not likely to result in a big rise in blood sugar. (Remember, we don't want food to hit your blood stream quickly, otherwise you're just going to feel hungry again shortly after.)

These are based on the *American Journal of Nutrition's* international table of glycemic index and glycemic load values: Meat, poultry, fish, avocados, salad vegetables, cheese, and eggs.

Tip 3: Go Nuts!

An ounce of nuts is a perfect healthy snack. An ounce of most nuts will add about 170 calories, 7 grams of carbs, 6 grams of protein, and 15 grams fat. (The higher amount of fat in nuts will take longer to digest and will help the snack seem more satisfying.)

- Hazelnuts and almonds are lowest in saturated fat
- Macadamia and hazelnuts are highest in monounsaturated fat (this is a very good thing)
- Pistachios and macadamia nuts are highest in fiber (about 3 grams per ounce)
- Walnuts have the most omega-3 fatty acids (also a very good thing)

Tip 4: Calling All Yogurt Fans

A container of light fruit yogurt (low fat and with artificial sweeteners) is a great snack at work or on the go. A 7-ounce container has about 13 grams of available carbohydrate and a glycemic index of 20, adding up to a glycemic load of only 2! Remember Tip #2 about the benefits of slow-release foods? Add some fresh fruit, ground flaxseed, or reduced-fat granola to yogurt to make a fun snack parfait!

Tip 5: Portable Fruit

Fruit can travel well in your car or briefcase and comes in handy for a quick pick-me-up, many offering just enough carbohydrates with a nice dose of fiber. You can make a more balanced snack by enjoying your fruit with cottage cheese, yogurt, or some cereal and milk.

The following fruits have a low glycemic load (5 or less per 4 ¼ oz. serving): Cherries, Grapefruit, Kiwi fruit, Oranges, Peaches, Pears, Plums, Cantaloupe, and Strawberries.

Tip 6: Get Your Whole Grain Snacks

The latest research suggests that people who eat whole grains have the lowest incidence of diabetes. They appear to increase the efficiency of insulin so that less is required to metabolize the sugar.

Tip 7: Eat Your Veggies

Cut up fresh, raw vegetables and serve them with a light ranch dressing, or with peanut butter, reduced fat cheese, or cottage cheese. Look past the basic salad greens and baby carrots and try jicama sticks (a refreshing, crispy white root), zucchini coins, bell pepper rings, or lightly cooked and chilled snow pea pods or green beans.

Tip 8: Try Trail Mix

The dried fruits in trail mix give you some fiber and carbohydrate calories, plus the nuts help round the snack off with protein, fat, and some more fiber. (Tip: Stay away from those that include ingredients such as sesame sticks or dried banana chips that may contain trans-containing hydrogenated oils. If you choose a trail mix with chocolate chips or M&Ms, just make sure there is just a sprinkling).

Tip 9: Don't Shovel Down Your Snack

Snacks need to be eaten slowly, too, just like meals. Don't forget that it takes 20 minutes for your brain to get the message that you are full. Give that message time to work before you decide the snack didn't do the trick. Make a point of enjoying a flavored mineral water (the unsweetened, no-calorie kind) at the same time. This will help you eat the snack slower, too.

Tip 10: Don't Make Your Snack a Meal

Snacks should be around 150-200 calories -- just enough energy to tide you over until your next meal, but not so much that it contributes as many calories as a meal. Try half of a whole-wheat bagel toasted with a slice of reduced fat cheddar instead of the whole bagel (150 calories vs. 300). Or try a cup of minestrone soup instead of a big bowl for a snack (150 calories vs. 300).[23]

And don't forget to account for all the calories you've already eaten that day. If you consumed a lot of calories high-calorie foods earlier, then skip your snack at night. If you consumed a low amount of calories, you probably still have room for another low-calorie snack.

Today's Challenge

Today I challenge you to choose healthy snacks over high calorie, nutrient deficient snacks. The food you eat should benefit your body not damage it. Stay conscious and focused on your goal to living a healthier lifestyle. You're just 10 days away from the body you deserve!

Day 11 Affirmation

"Beloved, I pray that you may prosper in all things and be in health, just as your soul prospers."

John 3:1-2

WHAT DID YOU LEARN FROM TODAY'S READING AND WHAT DID YOU LEARN ABOUT YOURSELF?

_____
_____
_____
_____
_____
_____
_____
_____
_____
_____
_____

HOW WILL YOU TAKE ONE STEP TOWARDS LIVING A HEALTHIER LIFESTYLE TODAY?

_____
_____
_____
_____
_____
_____
_____
_____
_____
_____
_____

LIST THREE THINGS (ANY THING)YOU'RE PROUD OF
YOURSELF FOR TODAY AND EXPLAIN WHY:

_____

_____

_____

_____

_____

_____

_____

_____

_____

_____

_____

_____

_____

_____

_____

_____

_____

SPEND FIVE MINUTES TODAY RECONNECTING YOUR
SPIRIT TO GOD. WRITE IT, PRAY IT OR SHOW IT!

_____

_____

_____

_____

_____

_____

_____

_____

_____

_____

_____

_____

_____

_____

_____

_____

Day 12
Vegetables: They're Not Just For Sunday Anymore

When I was a child, the best part of Sunday wasn't necessarily going to church, although I must admit it was fun watching the older church ladies "catch the spirit" and run around the church shoutin' and falling out on the floor. Wigs cocked to the side, slips showing, shoes left in the dust from too much Holy Ghost jumpin', the entertainment value alone was worth the trip! No, for me the best part of Sunday was the walk to Grandma's house after church and the dinner that would follow promptly at five o'clock. My Grandparents lived about half a mile from the church they helped build, the church I grew up in. They were very active members, always involved in church functions and ministries. Grandma served as an Usher and on the hospitality ministry and belonged to the local chapter of the Eastern Star. Grandpa served as a Deacon and belonged to the local Masonic chapter. Needless to say, we went to church a lot!

On days when the weather was nice, my Grandparents would often walk to church. I loved to walk home with them, all decked out in our Sunday best, Grandpa in his black suit, his Fedora tilted slightly to the side (Grandpa was smooth like that), and Grandma dressed like the woman of God she was in a modest blue dress adorned with a favorite brooch, the ensemble made complete with a hat, the good pocketbook (filled with hard candy and Kleenex for the kids) and white gloves. I would skip ahead or hold Grandpa's hand and enjoy the sights and sounds that created a lasting, warm memory I'll always cherish.

Grandma usually started dinner in the morning before she went to church. She would make whatever desserts we were going to have that day, peel and cut the potatoes, make the rolls, cornbread or both and put the meat in the oven on low so it would cook while she was gone. After church was when the maestro skillfully orchestrated the pots and pans into the rich, soulful symphony that we called Sunday dinner. While Grandma was putting the finishing touches on dinner I would set the dining room table, Sunday dinner was always a formal affair, lace tablecloth and all. Plates, glasses and silverware…check! Grandpa's extra large sweet tea glass in its place at the head of the table…check! Salt and pepper shakers at both ends of the table…check! Napkins folded in perfect triangles tucked under the plate on the right hand side…check! The table was all set for the parade of food that would be ushered in from the kitchen with a single call, "Dinner's ready!"

Sunday dinner is a tradition in the black family that has been passed down from generation to generation so I know I don't need to go into detail about the menu because you were there! You know that corn on-the-cob, fresh green beans, collard greens, sweet potatoes, mashed potatoes, okra, cabbage and carrots are a given. And black eyed-peas or red beans, peas, beets, squash and vegetables from the garden like tomatoes, onions and peppers made regular appearances at Sunday dinner. The table was a cornucopia of colors and aromas. Sunday dinner brought the family together for a feast to celebrate good fortune, good health and a good God.

Then, as if someone changed the channel and all of a sudden we're watching another show, Monday comes, and it's back to Hamburger Helper and light bread. Whoa! Wait a minute, what happened to all the vegetables? Where did the cornucopia of colors go? I like colors! Now don't get me wrong, there's nothing wrong with a little Hamburger Helper every now and then, but can I get a side of corn, green beans or a salad to go with it too?! How about some of those vitamin rich collards or fiber rich sweet potatoes? Sunday dinners are special, and for good reason, but when it comes to our health and the battle we're fighting against chronic disease, we have to take what we learned at the Sunday dinner table and apply it to the way we eat the rest of the week too. There's no better or easier way to reduce your risk of chronic disease and lose weight than by reducing the amount of fat, sodium and sugar in your diet and eating more fruits and vegetables.

Why Do We Need Vegetables

Research shows that fruits and vegetables are critical to promoting good health. They contain essential vitamins, minerals, and fiber that may help protect you from chronic diseases. Compared with people who consume a diet with only small amounts of fruits and vegetables, those who eat more generous amounts as part of a healthful diet are more likely to have reduced risk of chronic diseases including stroke, Type II diabetes, obesity, high blood pressure, heart disease and certain cancers. And, if that wasn't enough, you'll have more energy and look and feel better too!

The Colors of Health

You couldn't ask for more attractive packaging than the beautiful colors, shapes and sizes of fruits and vegetables, but their real beauty lies in what's inside. Fruits and vegetables are great sources of many vitamins, minerals and other natural substances. So to get a healthy variety, think color. Eating fruits and vegetables of different colors gives your body a wide range of valuable nutrients, like fiber, folate, potassium, and vitamins A and C. Some examples include green spinach, orange sweet potatoes, black beans, yellow corn, purple plums, red watermelon, and white onions. Explore your grocery store's produce department and introduce a new fruit or vegetable to your diet once a month. It's a great way to get the kids involved too!

How Many Fruits and Vegetables Do You Need Each Day

Every woman's need is different and is based on things like weight, age, and physical activity level. The CDC has a simple chart to help make sure you're getting enough fruits and vegetables in your daily meal plan.

	AGE	FRUITS	VEGETABLES
Less Active	19-30	2 cups	2 ½ cups
	31-50	1 ½ cups	2 ½ cups
	51+	1 ½ cups	2 cups
Moderately Active	19-50	2 cups	2 ½ cups
	51+	1 ½ cups	2 ½ cups
Active	19-50	2 cups	3 cups
	51+	2 cups	2 ½ cups

Here are some examples of what counts as a cup or half a cup of fruits and vegetables.

1 Cup	½ Cup
1 large ear of corn	5 pieces of broccoli
1 large orange	16 grapes
1 large sweet potato	4 large strawberries
1 small apple	1 small banana
1 medium grapefruit	6 baby carrots
1 cup cooked greens or spinach	1 large plum
2 stalks of celery	½ of a medium grapefruit

When you see it like this, you realize it's not impossible to increase your daily intake up to the recommended levels. An easy way to get the nutrition you need is to replace high calorie low nutrition snacks like cookies, candy or chips with nutrient rich, low calorie fruits and vegetables. Remember the old saying, an apple a day keeps the doctor away? It's true! A diet full of fruits and vegetables provides the necessary fiber to keep your digestive system running smoothly.

How to Use Fruits and Vegetables to Help Manage Your Weight

Using more fruits and vegetables along with whole grains and lean meats, nuts, and beans is a safe and healthy way to maintain weight loss or help you shed those unwanted pounds. We've already learned that in order to lose weight you have to eat fewer calories than your body uses. But that doesn't necessarily mean you have to eat less food! The water and fiber in fruits and vegetables will add bulk to your meals without adding unwanted calories. Your appetite will be satisfied and you will feel full longer.

Take a good look at your dinner plate. Vegetables, fruit, and whole grains should take up the largest portion of your plate. If they do not, cut back on some of the meat, white pasta, or rice. Add more beans, steamed broccoli, asparagus, greens, salad, or another favorite vegetable. This will reduce the total calories in your meal without reducing the amount of food you eat.

Snack Healthier

Instead of a high-calorie snack from a vending machine, bring some cut-up vegetables or fruit from home. One snack-sized bag of corn chips (1 ounce) has the same number of calories as a small apple, 1 cup of whole strawberries, AND 1 cup of carrots with ¼ cup of low-calorie dip!

Here are some examples of 100 calorie snacks that don't come in a box!
- a medium-size apple (72 calories)
- a medium-size banana (105 calories)
- 1 cup steamed green beans (44 calories)
- 1 cup blueberries (83 calories)
- 1 cup grapes (100 calories)

- 1 cup carrots (45 calories), broccoli (30 calories), or bell peppers (30 calories) with 2 tbsp. Hummus (46 calories)[24]

So what have we learned today? Fruits and vegetables help reduce your risk for chronic disease, they help replace vitamins and minerals your body is lacking, we should be eating a variety of colors, they are a good source of fiber and antioxidants, they boost your energy levels, and are important in controlling weight gain. Don't let vegetables be a Sunday dinner thing in your household; embrace vegetables, fall in love with fruit and watch your body reap the benefits!

Today's Challenge

Today I challenge you to make eating fruits and vegetables part of your daily meal plan 365 days a year. Also, if you haven't done it already, take some time today to boost your energy level and burn calories with exercise.

Day 12 Affirmation

"Lord, your discipline is good, for it leads to life and health. You restore my health and allow me to live!"

Isaiah 38:16

WHAT DID YOU LEARN FROM TODAY'S READING AND WHAT DID YOU LEARN ABOUT YOURSELF?

_____

_____

_____

_____

_____

_____

_____

_____

_____

_____

_____

_____

HOW WILL YOU TAKE ONE STEP TOWARDS LIVING A HEALTHIER LIFESTYLE TODAY?

_____

_____

_____

_____

_____

_____

_____

_____

_____

_____

_____

LIST THREE THINGS (ANY THING)YOU'RE PROUD OF YOURSELF FOR TODAY AND EXPLAIN WHY:

_____
_____
_____
_____
_____
_____
_____
_____
_____
_____
_____
_____
_____
_____
_____
_____

SPEND FIVE MINUTES TODAY RECONNECTING YOUR SPIRIT TO GOD. WRITE IT, PRAY IT OR SHOW IT!

_____
_____
_____
_____
_____
_____
_____
_____
_____
_____
_____
_____
_____
_____

Day 13
It's All About Me

Someone once said, "We are the sum of our experiences." Meaning, everything that has happened in our lives up to this point, makes us who we are right now at this very moment. Wow! Have you ever thought about it like that? When I think back over my life and all the experiences I've had, I know that this statement is true. I wouldn't be the woman I am today were it not for everything I've been through. Good times, bad times and times I'd wished God would take me from this earth right now. Sickness, health, weight gain, weight loss. I can look back at these experiences now with a smile and think that as hard as it may have been at the time, I'm still here!

If I am the sum of my experiences, who am I? I am the little girl who was teased at school for being taller than *everyone* else. I am the child who lost her father to cancer at age nine. I am the rebellious teenager always seeking my next adventure. I am the young woman who survived an abusive marriage, but still manages to love unconditionally. I am a proud mother because of the gift God gave me 23 years ago and I am a strong, God-fearing, black woman because of the strong, God-fearing, black women who came before me. I am truly the sum of my experiences and I've embraced every one of them with forgiveness and love. It's because of them that I am a stronger, more loving, caring, powerful, exciting woman today!

You are also the sum of your experiences. Today I want you to tell me who you are by answering a few questions. You can write them down or answer them in your head, but spend a few minutes really thinking about each of them. Ready? Tell me who you are.

1. What do you consider to be the defining moments of your life? The experiences that make you who you are today?

2. Have you let these experiences empower you or diminish you?

3. Do you see a correlation between these experiences and your body image? If yes, how has it affected your ability to maintain your ideal weight?

4. What can you do going forward to embrace your past, move forward and create a life that honors the woman you are right now?

5. Write a sentence, a paragraph or a poem about the woman you are today and what she means to you.

Today's Challenge

Today I challenge you to meditate on what was revealed to you today in your answers. You might be the sum of your experiences but you have a choice of whether you use those experiences to empower you or hold you hostage. Today I challenge you to release negativity and speak life into your spirit with positive, affirming, loving words. I love you and all that you are!

Day 13 Affirmation

"Jesus Christ is the same yesterday, today, and forever."
Hebrews 13:8

WHAT DID YOU LEARN FROM TODAY'S READING
AND WHAT DID YOU LEARN ABOUT YOURSELF?

_____
_____
_____
_____
_____
_____
_____
_____
_____
_____
_____
_____

HOW WILL YOU TAKE ONE STEP TOWARDS LIVING A
HEALTHIER LIFESTYLE TODAY?

_____
_____
_____
_____
_____
_____
_____
_____
_____
_____
_____
_____

LIST THREE THINGS (ANY THING) YOU'RE PROUD OF
YOURSELF FOR TODAY AND EXPLAIN WHY:

_____

_____

_____

_____

_____

_____

_____

_____

_____

_____

_____

_____

_____

_____

_____

_____

_____

_____

SPEND FIVE MINUTES TODAY RECONNECTING YOUR
SPIRIT TO GOD. WRITE IT, PRAY IT OR SHOW IT!

_____

_____

_____

_____

_____

_____

_____

_____

_____

_____

_____

_____

_____

_____

_____

Day 14
Do What? I Just Got My Hair Done!

Picture it! It's June, 1970 and the entire Smith-Marchbanks family is headed to Leavenworth, Kansas for a wedding. That's right, Leavenworth. This small farming community famous for its ties to the military and its federal prison, is the hometown of the woman my uncle is about to marry. They met while completing their undergraduate degrees at Kansas State University; he was a star basketball player and she a top sprinter on the track team. I'll never forget the day he brought her home to meet the family. It was like God had opened up the sky and dropped an angel on my Grandparents front porch. She was absolutely gorgeous! Flawless maple brown skin, coke bottle figure, the most perfect curly afro you'd ever seen and beautiful hazel eyes. She was everything I didn't know I wanted to be as a child of seven years old. I followed her around like a puppy and hung on her every word. I wanted to wear my hair like hers, I wanted to dress like her, and I wanted a cute, country accent like her. Pretty much I wanted to click my heels three times and be transported back to Kansas for a makeover because apparently that's where God did his best work! My uncle and his fiancée were a match made in heaven and the whole family was overjoyed when they announced their engagement.

From purple mountains majesty to amber waves of grain, the road trip from Pueblo, Colorado to Leavenworth, Kansas would take us thirteen hours, but no one was concerned about the distance; we were going to a wedding! The buzz of anticipation grew as the cars were loaded with everything we needed for the long trip. Games, books, pillows and snacks.

Coolers filled with ice, pop and Grandma's fried chicken brought extra weight to the cars trunks. The caravan of freshly washed cars would depart my Grandparents' house at dawn and travel the six hours it took to cross the border into the land of OZ before stopping at a rest area for a much needed potty break and picnic lunch. This was my first trip to Kansas during the summer months, so you can imagine my surprise when my brother opened the car door to let us out. Like a hot, wet blanket, the humid air wrapped itself around my body and choked my lungs till I gasped for air. I asked my Dad, "What is wrong with the air out here?" He just laughed and told me, "This is what it feels like with humidity in the air." It was hard for me to imagine having this sticky, wet covering on my skin every day and I couldn't wait to get back into the car in the comfort of the cool air conditioning.

Fast forward to the day of the wedding. With the men in one house and the women in another, it's time to get ready for the big event. I remember sitting at the kitchen table early that Saturday morning watching the ladies get their hair done. One by one they would sit in the chair by the stove for a quick touch-up around the edges with the hot comb or a tightening of the curls with the Marcel iron. Just as I was about to get up and leave I heard Grandma say, "Alright Karrie, your turn." I raised my eyebrows in disbelief, was I about to get *my* hair done?! I knew my cousin and I were flower girls in the wedding, but I didn't know I would be sporting a new doo for the occasion too! Thirty minutes, one singed ear and two hand slaps later I had perfectly pressed hair, curled bangs, locks down my back and a yellow bow in my hair! Wow! I couldn't believe the transformation. No more "naps" for me! Now I was bouncin' and behavin' just like the women in the commercials. I could hardly wait to complete the look with my yellow and white flower girl dress and white shoes.

I strutted around the house tossing my head from side to side trying to make my curls bounce, my brothers laughing, telling me I was going to give myself whiplash if I didn't stop. But I didn't care; I could hardly wait for everyone to see my new look! In fact, I was so excited I convinced my cousin to come outside with me (despite the fact that we had just been told not to) so we could practice our walk one more time. To make a long story short by leaving out the violence that ensued once my mother discovered us running around outside in the humidity, all of the perfect little spiral curls my grandmother had just spent time creating, had been magically transformed into something that made us look more like Buckwheat than Shirley Temple! I mean, who knew?! I was eight; I didn't understand the science of black hair versus humidity. All I knew was that Grandma was hotter than fish grease! Fortunately for us, Dr. Green didn't make a house call that day. There wasn't any time for all that, and it was just too doggone hot anyway! Side note: For those of you who didn't come from a family that believed in corporal punishment, Dr. Green was the name of the switch the elders in my family used to spank us with. Dr. Green had the medicine for whatever ailed you!

Needless to say, that experience was the beginning of the end of my freedom as a black female. From that day forward, I understood what it meant when women said, "Do what? I just got my hair done!" Because getting your "hair done" meant that someone had just spent hours washing, combing out, twisting, pressing and curling your hair, and you weren't about to mess it up! Getting your "hair done" meant that play time was over. Every activity that required you to sweat was now completely out of the question! Getting your "hair done" was also a rite of passage, just like a little boy's first trip to the barber shop. For us, going from twists or braids securely held with 5 different colors of barrettes to pressed or relaxed hair meant you were no longer a little girl, you were a young lady and young ladies *always* took care of their hair.

I conducted an impromptu survey of about 40 women and asked the question, "Name one thing a black woman won't do because she just had her hair done." Here are the top five answers.

1. Swimming - Waist high only; can't risk messing up the hair.
2. Sex -Ten minutes max and if they sweat on you or grab your hair, time's up!
3. Exercise - Only if it doesn't make you sweat.
4. Ride in a car with the windows down - If I want a breeze I'll turn the air on.
5. Dancing - One song limit unless you're wearing a wig or weave, but if you start to sweat its over!

It's a wonder we even move around at all! I mean seriously?! It's like black women have sweat-o-meters built into the tops of their heads and at the first sign of moisture all activity comes to a halt. Perhaps if we sweat when we ate we would put the fork down too! Ladies, isn't it about time we stop making excuses about our hair when it comes to our health? Remember the chronic disease list? Diet and lack of exercise were the leading causes *and* the easiest ways to reverse the effects of chronic disease. I understand a woman's hair is her glory and I know how much money you spent on that weave, but nobody will be looking at your hair when you're lying in a casket dead from a stroke! Okay, maybe at a black funeral they will, I mean I would, I'm just sayin'! But seriously, all kidding aside. Unless you've graced the cover of a magazine, have your own TV show, recording contract, or just hit Mega Ball, there is no personal trainer waiting at home to motivate you to exercise, and there is no personal chef in the kitchen cooking healthy meals for you and your family. Only *you* can decide it's time to take back your body and live a healthier lifestyle. So I dare you, ask yourself the following questions and if your answer is "Yes" to any of them, perhaps it's time you had a "come to Jesus meetin'" before you end up meetin' Jesus for real!

1. Am I letting my hair determine the size of my waistline?

2. Is my hair coming between me and the freedom to experience life to the fullest?

3. Do I spend more time and money on my hair than I do on healthy eating and exercise?

As black women, our desire to look good shouldn't stop at the neck. You can't buy good health like you buy good hair, but you *can* maintain the gift of health God has given you. Incorporating exercise into your daily routine doesn't mean you have to start training for a marathon. Nor does it mean you have to get all buff and look like a man. Start by walking every day, or do basic exercises like the ones you used to do in high school gym class. A quick ten minute workout every day will get your heart rate up, help you burn calories and tone and sculpt your body. And won't it be great when your body looks as good as your hair?!

Ten Minute Workout*

Do 60 seconds of each of the following exercises.

- Crunches
- Lunges
- Jumping jacks
- Push-ups (do a modified version on your knees if you have to)
- Squats
- Windmills (stand up with feet apart, arms out to the side. Touch the left foot with your right hand, stand up and do the other side.)

- High knee raises
- Side leg lifts
- Arm circles (forward 30 seconds, then backwards 30 sec.)
- Boxing punches

If you haven't exercised in awhile this ten minute workout might seem impossible to you at first, and you'll probably be a little sore the next day, but don't give up! Just do each exercise to the best of your ability and I promise you will get stronger every time you do the workout. Think about it, if we spent half the amount of time it takes to get our hair done working out, chronic disease for black women would be a thing of the past!

*Before starting any exercise program, check with your physician first.

Today's Challenge

Today I challenge you to choose your health over your hair and make exercise part of your lifestyle change. Be conscious of the hours you sit each day and vow to balance it out by being more active. Today I challenge you to move more and sit less.

Day 14 Affirmation

"Therefore know that the LORD your God, He is God, the faithful
God who keeps covenant and mercy for a thousand generations with
those who love Him and keep His commandments."

Deuteronomy 7:9

WHAT DID YOU LEARN FROM TODAY'S READING AND WHAT DID YOU LEARN ABOUT YOURSELF?

_____

_____

_____

_____

_____

_____

_____

_____

_____

_____

HOW WILL YOU TAKE ONE STEP TOWARDS LIVING A HEALTHIER LIFESTYLE TODAY?

_____

_____

_____

_____

_____

_____

_____

_____

_____

_____

LIST THREE THINGS (ANY THING)YOU'RE PROUD OF
YOURSELF FOR TODAY AND EXPLAIN WHY:

_____

_____

_____

_____

_____

_____

_____

_____

_____

_____

_____

_____

_____

_____

_____

SPEND FIVE MINUTES TODAY RECONNECTING YOUR
SPIRIT TO GOD. WRITE IT, PRAY IT OR SHOW IT!

_____

_____

_____

_____

_____

_____

_____

_____

_____

_____

_____

_____

_____

_____

Day 15
I Can't Lose Weight; I've Got a Slow Metabolism

Would you believe me if I told you it's difficult for some women to lose weight because their metabolism is slow? Of course you would! You're living proof, right? You've tried pills, exercise, meal plans that promise if you eat their food it will boost your metabolism, even starving yourself and you still can't lose weight. In fact, you're tired of watching your skinny friend eat all she wants while you sit there with celery sticks and water. Watch your mouth now, there's no name calling in this book! We love her like a sister; we just can't stand her with her boney behind! Well, what if I said you were wrong? What if I told you your metabolism is only a small part of the reason why you can't lose weight? And what if I told you good old fashioned healthy eating and exercise is all you need to lose your unwanted pounds? Before you throw this book in the trash, I've got a little science for you, so read on!

What is Metabolism?

While it's true that metabolism is linked to weight, it's not in the way you think. In fact, contrary to popular belief, a slow metabolism is rarely the cause of excess weight gain. Although your metabolism influences your body's basic energy needs, it's your food and beverage intake and your physical activity that ultimately determine how much you weigh. Highlight that last sentence for me; I want to make sure you got that.

By definition, **metabolism is simply the process by which your body converts the food you eat and drink into**

the energy your body needs to fuel you. Even when you're at rest, your body needs energy for bodily functions such as breathing, circulating blood, adjusting hormone levels, and growing and repairing cells. The number of calories your body uses to carry out these basic functions is known as your **basal metabolic rate** — what you might call metabolism. Your basal metabolic rate accounts for about 60 to 75 percent of the calories you burn every day.

Several factors that determine your individual basal metabolic rate include:

- **Your body size and composition.** Women who are overweight may actually have a higher metabolic rate than a woman who weighs much less simply because she weighs more. An overweight body has to work harder to perform the daily functions of circulating blood, breathing, digesting food, etc. so the metabolic rate is higher. Likewise, women who have more muscle mass (your skinny friend who eats everything) may have a higher metabolic rate because muscle burns more calories than fat.

- **Your age.** Starting at about age 25 our metabolic rate decreases 5 -10% per decade. As you get older, the amount of muscle you have tends to decrease, and fat becomes the majority of your weight. And what did we just learn? Muscle burns more calories than fat so if you're over 40 and gaining weight you're most likely losing muscle as well.[25]

In addition to your basal metabolic rate, two other factors determine how many calories your body burns each day:

Metabolism and Weight Gain

While it's easy to blame your metabolism for weight gain, metabolism is a natural process, and your body balances it to meet your individual needs. That's why when you go on the latest starvation diet, your body goes into survival mode and **slows the bodily processes** to conserve calories. Wow! Did you get that ladies? Did you ever think that the diet you're on could be the very thing that's keeping you from losing weight? Ever wonder what would happen if you stopped dieting and changed your eating habits to live a healthier lifestyle? I'm going to let that sink in for a minute because it's too important to miss. It's time to stop blaming our metabolism for our inability to lose weight and consider the real problem -- what we eat and how much we exercise. It's that simple, if you want to lose weight you have to eat fewer calories, increase the number of calories you burn through physical activity, or both. The more active you are, the more calories you burn, and the more fat you lose -- period.

Exercise and Your Metabolism

Here are some easy ways to increase your activity level and burn more calories:

- **Regular aerobic exercise.** Aerobic exercise is the most efficient way to burn calories and includes activities such as walking, bicycling, swimming or any cardio type fitness program. To keep your body healthy, you should do at least 30 minutes of physical activity every day. Get up off the couch in the evenings and walk the dog. No dog? Walk yourself! Or, blow the dust off the Wii you got last Christmas and start using it! If you're trying to lose weight, you may need to increase the amount of time or incorporate weights into your routine. If you can't make time for a longer workout, try 10-minute chunks of activity throughout the day. Remember, the more active you are, the quicker you'll start to see results.

- **Strength training.** Strength training exercises, such as weightlifting, are important because they help counteract muscle loss associated with aging. And since muscle tissue burns more calories than fat tissue does, muscle mass is a key factor in weight loss.

- **Lifestyle activities.** Any extra movement helps burn calories. Look for ways to walk and move around a few minutes more each day than the day before. Taking the stairs more often or walking the mall on your lunch hour are simple ways to burn more calories. Even activities such as cutting the grass, washing your car and housework burn calories and contribute to weight loss.

Stop the Slow Down

There are three easy things you can do right now to minimize the amount your metabolic rates decreases over the years:

- **Build Muscle** - Putting on lean muscle mass will increase the amount of calories you burn. Go back to that 10 minute workout I gave you and start doing it!
- **Eat Often** – Eating every 2 to 3 hours feeds muscle and starves fat. How? By keeping your body from going into starvation mode. When you skip meals you train your body to store fat.
- **Eat Right** – Eating every 2 to 3 hours doesn't mean a handful of cookies, chips or a candy bar. Instead, eat foods high in protein (lean meat, fish, eggs, nuts, protein shakes) and fiber (flaxseed, fruits and vegetables). Your body has to work hard to break down these nutrients therefore, increasing the amount of calories burned. Start taking two healthy snacks to work with you to fill the gaps between lunch and dinner.

No Magic Pill

Although it's easy to get sucked into the latest infomercial on fat burning supplements, don't believe the hype! Dietary supplement manufacturers aren't required by the Food and Drug Administration to prove that their products are safe or effective. Some products that claim to speed up your metabolism may cause undesirable or even dangerous side effects. [26] Be careful ladies and remember, God gave you *one* body, that's all you get, you can either nourish and protect it or abuse it and watch it wither away. I believe you've already made your choice. Are you ready to take the next step?!

Today's Challenge

Today I challenge you to think about the excuses you've made to justify why you've let yourself go; and then ask yourself, are you letting those excuses define who you are? If the answer is yes, I challenge you to release yourself from that definition and come up with one that empowers and strengthens you. If the answer is no, read today's challenge again and this time, be honest with yourself!

Day 15 Affirmation

"I delight to do Your will, O my God! Indeed, Your law is written in my heart."

Psalm 40:8

WHAT DID YOU LEARN FROM TODAY'S READING AND WHAT DID YOU LEARN ABOUT YOURSELF?

_____

_____

_____

_____

_____

_____

_____

_____

_____

_____

_____

_____

_____

HOW WILL YOU TAKE ONE STEP TOWARDS LIVING A HEALTHIER LIFESTYLE TODAY?

_____

_____

_____

_____

_____

_____

_____

_____

_____

LIST THREE THINGS (ANY THING)YOU'RE PROUD OF YOURSELF FOR TODAY AND EXPLAIN WHY:

_____
_____
_____
_____
_____
_____
_____
_____
_____
_____
_____
_____
_____
_____
_____
_____

SPEND FIVE MINUTES TODAY RECONNECTING YOUR SPIRIT TO GOD. WRITE IT, PRAY IT OR SHOW IT!

_____
_____
_____
_____
_____
_____
_____
_____
_____
_____
_____
_____
_____
_____
_____
_____

Day 16
The "Baby's" Five, Let it Go

Early one Saturday morning, as I sat in the chair at the beauty salon and watched the frenzy of activity that's typical of a black beauty establishment, I smiled as I grabbed bits and pieces of conversations that traveled energetically through the air. I heard the latest gossip from the pews, learned about a boyfriend who was about to be kicked to the curb for cheating, and everyone, it seemed, had something to say about the latest Tyler Perry movie. No topic was too sensitive for these women; they had an answer to every problem or situation and didn't mind sharing their two cents about it either. My ears perked up when the conversation between two women sitting close by turned to weight loss. "Girl, it's hard to lose weight. I've tried every diet out there, and all they do is make me hungry!" the first woman said to the other. "I hear you girl! I gained thirty pounds with little Kevin, and I'm still trying to lose the weight," she replied. Now, being a mother myself, I knew exactly what she was talking about. I put on 40 pounds when I was pregnant with my daughter, so I was completely sympathetic to her struggle, that is, until little Kevin walks over to his mother and asks if he can have a quarter for the candy machine! "Boy, don't you see me talkin?" she says as she reaches into her purse and pulls out fifty cents. "Here Kevin, and bring me some too!"

Now, I don't know about you but I'm thinking this woman has a serious case of denial! Like a lot of women who struggle with weight loss, she was quick to transfer her issues with food away from herself and onto to someone else -- in this case her child. Some of us blame our husbands, money or the environment we live in, everything but ourselves. To listen to this woman talk about her "struggle" with losing her pregnancy weight, you would have thought she had just given birth a week ago! Okay, underline this next sentence. The words "baby fat" can no longer be applied to the 40 pounds you're still carrying around if you *and* the "baby" are eating the same food!

What excuse are you using to rationalize your extra pounds? Is it the kids? Your husband who won't exercise with you? Is it the cost of joining a gym that's keeping you fat? Lack of time? Or, is it all the food people bring in at the job? I've heard them all. Heck I used to say some of them! My favorite excuse for eating a Big Mac value meal went something like this, "I'll eat whatever I want today and tomorrow I'll just work it off!" Raise your hand if you think I made it to the gym the next day. Exactly! If I couldn't fool you, do you think I was fooling myself? Absolutely not! I knew exactly what I was doing when I ate that Big Mac, and I knew I would pay for it. I could feel my thighs expand with every bite and yet I did it anyway. So tell me, what will it take for you to stop living in denial and say, "Enough!"

Freedom from the Ups and Downs of Dieting

Raise your hand if you've tried more than one fad diet in your lifetime. Raise your hand if you've taken diet pills to lose weight. Now raise your hand, if after trying these methods, you didn't lose any weight or gained the weight back plus more! If you raised your hand to the last question, you're not alone. Research shows that 4 out of 5 people who lose weight on a strict diet plan will gain it back. Why? Now this is where you expect me to use big words and say something all doctorish about how fat cells multiply and grow back twice their size so you'll feel better about your inability to lose weight and keep it off. Sorry, it was denial that got you into this mess, only the truth will set you free! The truth is diets are designed to *restrict* you from eating certain things, carbs, fats, protein, etc., when in reality; your body needs all those things to stay healthy. I mean seriously, are you really going to eat hot dogs and boiled eggs every day for the rest of their life?! Who does that?! You might think your love for bread is enough to sustain you till the day you die, but I'm willing to bet that before the month is over your friends will find you huddled in the corner of a dark closet attacking a plate of meat and vegetables like a wild animal!

So, instead of denying our bodies of the nutrients they need, let's try something different this time. Are you with me? From this moment on you are not allowed to use the word "diet." Go ahead and remove it from your vocabulary because you won't need it anymore. Instead, we're going to start saying, "healthier lifestyle," because a healthier lifestyle is something everyone can achieve regardless of their age, kids, where they live, husband, how much time and money they have or where they work. You won't need an expensive gym membership or pricey mail order food to achieve a healthier lifestyle. All you need, all you've ever needed, is the belief that you are worth it.

Today's Challenge

Today I challenge you to truly **believe** that you are "fearfully and wonderfully made" (Psalm 139:14) and can accomplish anything you set your mind to -- even if it's losing weight. Someone once said, "We only ask for what we believe we deserve." You were born with the gift of health, are you so arrogant that you would deny yourself what God has already given you?! Today is the day you break away from denial and start living a healthier lifestyle. Why? Because *you deserve it!*

Sweet Tea & Cornbread

Day 16 Affirmation

"For God has not given us a spirit of fear, but of power and of love and of a sound mind."

2 Timothy 1:7

WHAT DID YOU LEARN FROM TODAY'S READING AND WHAT DID YOU LEARN ABOUT YOURSELF?

_____

_____

_____

_____

_____

_____

_____

_____

_____

_____

_____

HOW WILL YOU TAKE ONE STEP TOWARDS LIVING A HEALTHIER LIFESTYLE TODAY?

_____

_____

_____

_____

_____

_____

_____

_____

_____

_____

_____

LIST THREE THINGS (ANY THING) YOU'RE PROUD OF YOURSELF FOR TODAY AND EXPLAIN WHY:

_____

_____

_____

_____

_____

_____

_____

_____

_____

_____

_____

_____

_____

_____

_____

_____

SPEND FIVE MINUTES TODAY RECONNECTING YOUR SPIRIT TO GOD. WRITE IT, PRAY IT OR SHOW IT!

_____

_____

_____

_____

_____

_____

_____

_____

_____

_____

_____

_____

_____

_____

_____

_____

Day 17
A Size 20 is the New 6

When I decided enough was enough and started living a healthier lifestyle my friends thought I was either sick or crazy. Every time we went out to eat and I ordered something from the healthy side of the menu, heads would turn, and I would get the "what's up with you" look. If I said no to sharing buttered popcorn at the movies, I was a traitor, and when I turned down dessert after the movies, they almost voted me off the island, but as soon as I started to lose weight they all wanted to know what I was doing. (Funny how it didn't click in their minds just by watching the way I ate.) Convinced I must have found some new miracle drug, they didn't want to hear that I had made the decision to cut back on the amount of sugar, salt and fat I ate. "Well, if you don't want to tell us just say so!" was the response I got from some of them.

About a year later I got a call from one of my friends. She was frustrated and almost in tears as she told me how she had just come from shopping at the mall only to realize that she now fit comfortably in a size 20. She explained how at first she thought it was just the brand she was trying on, "You know how some designers switch up the sizes to make you think you're really bigger than you are when you haven't changed sizes at all?" She said, with as much confidence as she could. Annoyed with the selections at that particular store she left in search of a boutique that knew what "real women" looked like. She went from store to store trying on clothes until she just couldn't take it anymore and left the mall empty handed. "This is why I hate shopping; nothing fits and if it fits it doesn't look right!" she screamed into the phone. "I have nothing to wear and I'm tired of it!" she said, her voice trembling slightly. I could tell she was at the end of her rope so I asked her what she was going to do about it. "What do you mean?" she asked. "You said you were tired of it, did you mean shopping or being a size 20?" I asked, glad that I was on the other end of the phone and not close enough for her to snatch me up! "Oh, so you got jokes now?" she answered tartly. "You said it, not me, I'm just trying to figure out if there's any way I can help." "Would you?!" she said in a voice that was way too happy, and I knew instantly that I had just been played.

As she braced herself for the harsh diet she thought I was about to put her on, she listened incredulously when I explained that all she needed to do was listen to her body and start living a healthier lifestyle. As soon as her laughter quieted down, I asked her all the questions I've asked you in this book. I explained the difference between good carbs and bad, how to reduce her sodium intake and the benefit of eating more fruits and vegetables, then I told her what exercises to do for her body type. She asked me how long she had to do these things, and I explained that this wasn't some diet that you started and stopped, it was a lifestyle change. Unconvinced that she could go without her daily bag of peanut M&M's, and Mountain Dew, she told me she would give it three weeks which was exactly the amount of time before her next doctor's appointment.

In the beginning, sticking to the plan was difficult for her. She suffered from headaches due to a lack of caffeine and the decreased amounts of sugar she was ingesting. Needless to say, she was not a happy camper! I received a very interesting text message from her five days into her new lifestyle, which testified to her mental state: "Serving size, two tablespoons. Who the h@#! eats two tablespoons of ANYTHING?!" The following week she invited me over for dinner. I entered the house slowly, checking for boobie traps along the way to the kitchen. After inspecting the barstool for explosives, I took my seat at the counter and watched carefully as she prepared our meal. Baked chicken (lightly seasoned), steamed broccoli (no butter) and boiled sweet potatoes (sweetened with Splenda®) completed the menu for the evening. "What, no bread? No mashed potatoes and gravy?" I teased jokingly. "Don't even play like that -- not today." she said while gripping the knife in her hand a little too tightly for my comfort.

Three weeks to the day she called to give me her report. I could hear the excitement in her voice when she told me the story of how shocked her doctor was when she had taken her blood pressure. Her blood pressure numbers were so low the doctor checked them twice! And then the doctor told her she was taking her off the blood pressure medication as long as she continued to keep it under control. She went on to say she had lost 15 pounds and that after years of being on medication for diabetes, she was down from six shots a day to just two! She said she felt like a new woman and joked about having to buy new clothes. "Karrie," she said, "you've changed my life."

Today's Challenge

Today I challenge you to imagine what your life could be like without the extra weight, without the medications, without the aches and pains and then…put your big girl panties on and make it happen! I can't wait to hear your success stories!

Day 17 Affirmation

"So do not fear, for I am with you; do not be dismayed, for I am your God. I will strengthen you and help you; I will uphold you with my righteous right hand."

Isaiah 41:10

WHAT DID YOU LEARN FROM TODAY'S READING AND WHAT DID YOU LEARN ABOUT YOURSELF?

_____
_____
_____
_____
_____
_____
_____
_____
_____
_____
_____
_____

HOW WILL YOU TAKE ONE STEP TOWARDS LIVING A HEALTHIER LIFESTYLE TODAY?

_____
_____
_____
_____
_____
_____
_____
_____
_____
_____

LIST THREE THINGS (ANY THING)YOU'RE PROUD OF YOURSELF FOR TODAY AND EXPLAIN WHY:

_____

_____

_____

_____

_____

_____

_____

_____

_____

_____

_____

_____

_____

_____

_____

_____

SPEND FIVE MINUTES TODAY RECONNECTING YOUR SPIRIT TO GOD. WRITE IT, PRAY IT OR SHOW IT!

_____

_____

_____

_____

_____

_____

_____

_____

_____

_____

_____

_____

_____

_____

Day 18
Overweight and Undernourished

Overweight and undernourished, it sounds like an oxymoron, doesn't it? Well, unfortunately it's not. Too many black women fall into this category because of our poor eating habits and the lack of readily available fresh produce in some of our neighborhoods. We know from previous chapters that you don't gain weight by over indulging in fresh fruits and vegetables. You put on the pounds with fast food, processed foods and sugary drinks. These foods are loaded with empty calories and lack the nutrition your body needs to fight disease and function properly, and the result is a body that is overweight and undernourished.

Feeding your body the proper nutrition is vital if your goal is to lose weight and live a healthier lifestyle. Starvation diets do one thing --they starve your body of the nutrients it needs to maintain a healthy weight. That's it! The vitamins and minerals you get from eating whole foods (whole grains, fruits, vegetables, nuts) help your body fight chronic disease, increase energy, support immune function and help maintain healthy bones, skin, hair and nails. When your body is properly fed, you feel better on the inside and look better on the outside.

Can Taking Vitamins or Supplements Help?

There is no doubt the battle against chronic disease can be won with the proper diet and exercise. And there is no doubt the best way to get the nutrition you need is by eating whole foods, just the way God intended. But in today's frantic world it can be a struggle to eat all the vitamins and minerals your body needs every day from food. Taking vitamin supplements is a good way enhance your healthy lifestyle change by ensuring that your body is getting the nutrition it needs to keep you on the right track.

Not All Vitamins are Created Equal

If you're going to take a multivitamin or supplement, read the labels and make sure you're buying **whole food** vitamins. What's the difference? **Whole food vitamins and supplements are made from real foods.** They are more easily digested and are absorbed completely by your body. Synthetic vitamins are chemically produced; they don't contain any real food, are not absorbed completely and can cause nausea or upset stomach. So, how do you know if your vitamin brand is whole food or synthetic? Here's what to look for.

Actual Whole Food Vitamin C Label:

Supplement Facts

Serving Size: 2 Capsules
Servings Per Container: 30

	Amount Per Serving	%DV
Vitamin C (naturally occurring from Organic Gold Standard Amla [Emblica officinalis] and Citrus Fruits [Citrus limon, aurantium] and Acerola Cherry Fruit [Malpighia glabra])	500 mg	833%
Organic Gold Standard Amla (certified organic amla fruit)	1000 mg	+
Organic Whole Food Bioflavonoids (Quercetins, Rutin, Leucodelphinidin) from Organic Gold Standard Amla Berry	100 mg	+

Other Ingredients: Certified Organic Whole Food Blend [Organic Acerola Extract, Apple Fruit, Broccoli Sprout, Cauliflower Sprout, Collard, Cordyceps Mushroom Mycelia (Cordyceps sinensis), Kale, Kale Sprout, Maitake Mushroom Mycelia (Grifola frondosa), Nettle, Parsley, Pure Beet Juice, Pure Carrot Juice, Pure Spirulina, Reishi Mushroom Mycelia (Ganoderma lucidum), Shiitake Mushroom Mycelia (Lentinula edodes), Spinach, Tomato Juice, Wild Bilberry, Wild Blueberry, Wild Lingonberry, Pure Chlorella], Organic Rice Maltodextrin, Mineral Fatty Acid Esters (Ca, Mg) from Safflower.
Suggested Use: As a dietary supplement, two capsules daily.

Actual Synthetic C Vitamin Label:

Supplement Facts

Serving Size: 1 Vegetarian Capsule
Servings Per Container: 100

	Amount Per Serving	%DV
Vitamin C (as Ascorbic Acid)	2000 mg	3333%

Other Ingredients: Hydroxypropyl methylcellulose, microcrystalline cellulose, magnesium stearate. **Suggested Use:** 1 or 2 capsules with each meal, or as directed by a healthcare practitioner.

There are two things I want you to take note of. First, the whole food Vitamin C is made from naturally occurring fruits and vegetables. And secondly, the whole food vitamin doesn't have to be taken with a meal. Why? Because it is a meal! It's food your body recognizes and it's processed as such in order to give you the health benefits your body needs. Ascorbic Acid is not food; your body doesn't recognize it and can't process it. It has to be taken with food to keep from upsetting your stomach.

Which Vitamins Does Your Body Need for Optimum Health?

Before you go to your local superstore and buy a cart full of vitamins, talk to your doctor and find out what vitamin regimen is right for your body type. Because no two women's bodies are the same, no two vitamin regimens should be the same. Age, weight, physical activity level and your current state of health are factors in determining which vitamins will benefit you the most.

Here's a basic vitamin regimen for women. Check with your doctor for correct dosage.

1. Calcium/Magnesium
As women we need calcium to protect our bones from osteoporosis, as we age our bodies lose calcium and it must be replaced. Magnesium is added to protect you from constipation, bloating and other gastrointestinal discomforts caused by the calcium supplement. You can get calcium naturally by eating leafy green vegetables such as, collards, spinach and kale.

2. Vitamin D3
Vitamin D3 deficiency has been linked to joint pain, fatigue, high blood pressure, multiple sclerosis and some

cancers. Taking it also increases the absorption of calcium helping to strengthen your bones. You can get this vitamin naturally by increasing the amount of time you spend in the sun. Sunshine triggers your skin to produce Vitamin D naturally. But don't forget the sunscreen!

3. DHA

DHA omega-3 fatty acids are the good fats that help reduce clogging of the arteries and help increase healthy (HDL or "good") cholesterol numbers. They are naturally found in fish like salmon and tuna, so eat up!

4. Multivitamin

Taking a multivitamin is a good way to make sure your body is getting all the nutrients it needs. Look for whole-food multivitamins and if the label suggests taking two a day, take one in the morning and one at night. Why? Because multivitamins are usually water-soluble which means your body will release them in your urine within eight to 16 hours so by splitting the dose your body is getting the biggest bang for your buck!

5. Probiotics

Probiotics are a type of good bacteria that is naturally occurring in your body. In fact, you were born with it! They help regulate your digestive system and help your body fight infection and disease. Unfortunately, through poor eating habits and increased antibiotic use, our bodies are lacking the good bacteria and it must be replaced. Eating yogurt is a good way to increase the good bacteria in your body without taking supplements.

6. CoQ10

CoQ10 is crucial for heart health. As you age, your body

naturally makes less of this micronutrient, so supplements are vital to keep your heart healthy and strong. [27]

In addition to the supplements listed here, I'm going to add one of my personal favorites: Biotin. Biotin keeps your hair, skin and nails healthy and strong. I take 1000mcg in the morning and again at night.

Are you overweight and undernourished? Is your body lacking the nutrients it needs to get healthy and stay healthy? Is your body showing the signs of age and poor nutrition? Signs like hair loss, brittle finger and toe nails, bruises that won't go away, feeling tired, lack of energy, acne, or dull eyes? In order to take back your body and live a healthier lifestyle, you must first listen to your body. Hear what's it's telling you about your food choices. Then you must feed it what it needs to thrive -- healthy foods and exercise. Vitamin supplements will help you fill in the gaps and keep your body nourished and on the right track. The body you deserve is within reach ladies. Are you ready to take the next step?

Today's Challenge

Today I challenge you to recognize the difference between whole foods and the nutrient deficient foods you're currently eating. Give your body the nutrition it's craving and you will see it change right before your eyes. Guaranteed!

Day 18 Affirmation

"For assuredly, I say to you, whoever says to this mountain, 'Be removed and be cast into the sea,' and does not doubt in his heart, but believes that those things he says will be done, he will have whatever he says."

Mark 11:23

WHAT DID YOU LEARN FROM TODAY'S READING AND WHAT DID YOU LEARN ABOUT YOURSELF?

_____

_____

_____

_____

_____

_____

_____

_____

_____

_____

_____

HOW WILL YOU TAKE ONE STEP TOWARDS LIVING A HEALTHIER LIFESTYLE TODAY?

_____

_____

_____

_____

_____

_____

_____

_____

_____

LIST THREE THINGS (ANY THING)YOU'RE PROUD OF YOURSELF FOR TODAY AND EXPLAIN WHY:

_____
_____
_____
_____
_____
_____
_____
_____
_____
_____
_____
_____
_____
_____
_____
_____
_____

SPEND FIVE MINUTES TODAY RECONNECTING YOUR SPIRIT TO GOD. WRITE IT, PRAY IT OR SHOW IT!

_____
_____
_____
_____
_____
_____
_____
_____
_____
_____
_____
_____
_____
_____
_____
_____

Day 19
How to Read Labels

ealthy eating starts with knowing what you're putting in your mouth! Reading nutrition labels is the best way to know you're making healthier food choices. Nutrition facts on food labels can help you watch your weight and limit fat, sugar, or salt.

Nutrition Label Facts

Start here

Check the total calories per serving

Limit these nutrients

Get enough of these nutrients

Quick Guide to % Daily Value:
5% or less is low
20% or more is high

Nutrition Facts

Serving Size 1 slice (47g)
Servings Per Container 6

Amount Per Serving

Calories 160   Calories from Fat 90

	% Daily Value*
Total Fat 10g	15%
Saturated Fat 2.5g	11%
Trans Fat 2g	
Cholesterol 0mg	0%
Sodium 300mg	12%
Total Carb 15g	5%
Dietary Fiber less than 1g	3%
Sugars 1g	
Protein 3g	

Vitamin A 0%	Vitamin C 4%
Calcium 45%	Iron 0%
Thiamin 8%	Riboflavin 0%
Niacin 6%	

*Percent Daily Values are based on a 2,000 calorie diet. Your daily values may be higher or lower depending on your calorie needs.

- **Start here:** Note the size of a single serving and how many servings are in the package.
- **Check total calories per serving:** Look at the serving size and how many servings you're really consuming. If you double the servings you eat, you double the calories and nutrients, including the Percent Daily Value (% DV).
- **Limit these nutrients:** Remember, you need to limit your total fat to no more than 56–78 grams a day — including no more than 16 grams of saturated fat, less than two grams of trans fat, and less than 300 mg cholesterol (for a 2,000 calorie diet).
- **Get enough of these nutrients:** Make sure you get 100 percent of the fiber, vitamins and other nutrients you need every day.
- **Quick guide to % DV:** The % DV section tells you the percent of each nutrient in a single serving, in terms of the daily recommended amount. As a guide, if you want to consume less of a nutrient (such as saturated fat, cholesterol or sodium), choose foods with a lower % DV — 5 percent or less is low. If you want to consume more of a nutrient (such as fiber), seek foods with a higher % DV — 20 percent or more is high.

Remember that the information shown in these panels is based on 2,000 calories a day. You may need to consume less or more than 2,000 calories depending upon your age, gender, activity level, and whether you're trying to lose, gain or maintain your weight.[28]

The Truth About Labels

- **Fortified, enriched, added, extra, and plus.** This means nutrients such as minerals and fiber have been removed and vitamins added in processing. Look for 100% whole-wheat bread, and high-fiber, low-sugar cereals.

- **Fruit drink.** This means there's probably little or no real fruit and a lot of sugar. Instead, look for products that say "100% Fruit Juice."

- **Made with wheat, rye, or multigrains.** These products have very little whole grain. Look for the word "whole" before the grain to ensure that you're getting a 100 percent whole-grain product.

- **Natural.** The manufacturer started with a natural source, but once it's processed, the food may not resemble anything natural. Look for "100% All Natural" and "No Preservatives."

- **Organically grown, pesticide-free, or no artificial ingredients.** Trust only labels that say "Certified Organically Grown."

- **Sugar-free or fat-free.** Don't assume the product is low-calorie. The manufacturer compensated with unhealthy ingredients that don't taste very good and, here's the kicker, have no fewer calories than the real thing.[29]

Today's Challenge

Today I challenge you to get familiar with what you're feeding your body. Nutrition is important for maintaining a healthy weight, fighting disease and illness and slowing the aging process. Get comfortable with reading labels so you can choose the best foods for your body.

Day 19 Affirmation

"You have given me your shield of victory; your help has made me great." "You have made a wide path for my feet to keep them from slipping."

2 Samuel 22:36-38

WHAT DID YOU LEARN FROM TODAY'S READING AND WHAT DID YOU LEARN ABOUT YOURSELF?

_____

_____

_____

_____

_____

_____

_____

_____

_____

_____

_____

_____

HOW WILL YOU TAKE ONE STEP TOWARDS LIVING A HEALTHIER LIFESTYLE TODAY?

_____

_____

_____

_____

_____

_____

_____

_____

LIST THREE THINGS (ANY THING)YOU'RE PROUD OF YOURSELF FOR TODAY AND EXPLAIN WHY:

_____

_____

_____

_____

_____

_____

_____

_____

_____

_____

_____

_____

_____

_____

_____

_____

_____

SPEND FIVE MINUTES TODAY RECONNECTING YOUR SPIRIT TO GOD. WRITE IT, PRAY IT OR SHOW IT!

_____

_____

_____

_____

_____

_____

_____

_____

_____

_____

_____

_____

_____

_____

Day 20
Fiber Rich Foods List

S imply doubling the amount of fiber you eat from the average of 15 grams per day to around 30 grams helps reduce calorie intake by making you feel full longer. The American Dietetic Association recommends 20 grams to 35 grams of fiber a day. Women need about 25 grams of fiber a day for optimal health protection against chronic disease.

FRUIT	AMOUNT	TOTAL FIBER (grams)
Apples with skin	1 medium	**5.00**
Apricot	3 medium	0.98
Apricots, dried	5 pieces	2.89
Banana	1 medium	3.92
Blueberries	1 cup	4.18
Cantaloupe, cubes	1 cup	1.28
Figs, dried	2 medium	3.74
Grapefruit	1/2 medium	**6.12**
Orange, navel	1 medium	3.40
Peach	1 medium	2.00
Peaches, dried	3 pieces	3.18
Pear	1 medium	**5.08**
Plum	1 medium	1.00
Raisins	1.5 oz box	1.60
Raspberries	1 cup	**8.34**
Strawberries	1 cup	3.98

VEGETABLES	AMOUNT	TOTAL FIBER (grams)
Avocado (fruit)	1 medium	**11.84**
Beets, cooked	1 cup	2.85
Beet greens	1 cup	4.20
Broccoli, cooked	1 cup	4.50
Brussels sprouts	1 cup	2.84
Cabbage, cooked	1 cup	4.20
Carrot	1 medium	2.00
Carrot, cooked	1 cup	**5.22**
Cauliflower, cooked	1 cup	3.43
Cole slaw	1 cup	4.00
Collard greens, cooked	1 cup	2.58
Corn, sweet	1 cup	4.66
Green beans	1 cup	3.95
Celery	1 stalk	1.02
Kale, cooked	1 cup	**7.20**
Onions, raw	1 cup	2.88
Peas, cooked	1 cup	**8.84**
Peppers, sweet	1 cup	2.62
Pop corn, air-popped	3 cups	3.60
Potato, baked w/skin	1 medium	4.80
Spinach, cooked	1 cup	4.32
Summer squash, cooked	1 cup	2.52
Sweet potato, cooked	1 cup	**5.94**
Swiss chard, cooked	1 cup	3.68
Tomato	1 medium	1.00
Winter squash, cooked	1 cup	**5.74**
Zucchini, cooked	1 cup	2.63

CEREAL, GRAINS, PASTA	AMOUNT	TOTAL FIBER (grams)
Bran cereal	1 cup	**19.94**
Bread, whole wheat	1 slice	2.00
Oats, rolled dry	1 cup	**12.00**
Pasta, whole wheat	1 cup	**6.34**

Rice, dry brown	1 cup	**7.98**

BEANS, NUTS, SEEDS	AMOUNT	TOTAL FIBER (grams)
Almonds	1 oz	4.22
Black beans, cooked	1 cup	**14.92**
Cashews	1 oz	1.00
Flax seeds	3 tbs	**6.97**
Kidney beans, cooked	1 cup	**13.33**
Lentils, red cooked	1 cup	**15.64**
Lima beans, cooked	1 cup	**13.16**
Peanuts	1 oz	2.30
Pistachio nuts	1 oz	3.10
Pumpkin seeds	1/4 cup	4.12
Soybeans, cooked	1 cup	**7.62**
Sunflower seeds	1/4 cup	3.00
Walnuts	1 oz	3.08

Today's Challenge

Today I challenge you to increase the amount of fiber in your daily diet. Fiber helps you feel full longer so you're not as hungry when you're trying to lose weight and it improves the digestive process so your body runs smoothly.

Day 20 Affirmation

"Finally, brothers and sisters, whatever is true, whatever is noble, whatever is right, whatever is pure, whatever is lovely, whatever is admirable—if anything is excellent or praiseworthy—think about such things. Whatever you have learned or received or heard from me, or seen in me—put it into practice. And the God of peace will be with you."

Philippians 4:8

WHAT DID YOU LEARN FROM TODAY'S READING AND WHAT DID YOU LEARN ABOUT YOURSELF?

_____
_____
_____
_____
_____
_____
_____
_____
_____
_____
_____
_____

HOW WILL YOU TAKE ONE STEP TOWARDS LIVING A HEALTHIER LIFESTYLE TODAY?

_____
_____
_____
_____
_____
_____

_____

_____

_____

_____

_____

LIST THREE THINGS (ANY THING)YOU'RE PROUD OF
YOURSELF FOR TODAY AND EXPLAIN WHY:

_____

_____

_____

_____

_____

_____

_____

_____

_____

_____

_____

_____

_____

SPEND FIVE MINUTES TODAY RECONNECTING YOUR
SPIRIT TO GOD. WRITE IT, PRAY IT OR SHOW IT!

_____

_____

_____

_____

_____

_____

_____

_____

_____

_____

Day 21
Healthy Foods List

W e've learned that our diets should include fruits, vegetables, fiber, omega-3s, etc., but do you know which foods pack the most punch? This handy and informative healthy shopping list explains the impact certain foods have on our bodies and includes dozens of tasty food options to help you enjoy a healthy daily diet.

What to buy when you go to the store.

Cholesterol and Blood Sugar Helpers

Some foods rich in soluble fiber and/or plant sterols can help lower blood cholesterol levels, enhance digestive health and minimize the rise in blood sugar levels after a meal (good for diabetics)

Antioxidant Rich

Antioxidants help to prevent and repair damage done by free radicals in the environment. A diet rich in antioxidents may also enhance immunity and lower the risk of cancer. Antioxidants include some vitamins, minerals and flavanoids.

Cholesterol & Blood Sugar Helpers
- Vegetables
- Fruits
- Whole grains
- Beans
- Nuts
- Seeds

Foods Enriched with Plant Sterols
- Orange juice
- Yogurts
- Margarines
- Cereal
- Granola
- chocolate

Omega 3 Fatty Acid Rich Foods
- Salmon
- Lake trout

High Fiber
- Most vegetables
- Pears
- Mangoes
- Kiwi
- Plums
- Blackberries
- Raspberries
- Peaches
- Strawberries
- Apples
- Citrus fruits
- Dried fruits
- Nuts, seeds
- Dried peas
- Beans
- Lentils
- Whole grains
- Oatmeal
- Oat bran

Antioxident Rich
- artichokes
- russet potatoes
- apples
- blueberries
- blackberries
- cherries
- cranberries
- raspberries
- strawberries
- plums
- prunes
- pecans
- small red beans
- kidney beans
- pinto beans
- black beans
- coffee
- red wine
- tea

High Fiber

There are two kinds of fiber, soluable and insoluable, both are important for a healthy digestive system. Additionally, insoluable fiber adds bulk to the diet which is helpful for weight control. A diet high in both fibers can reduce the risk of heart disease and diabetes.

Low Sodium

Eating foods high in sodium may cause high blood pressure. Lower your consumption of high sodium foods and eat foods rich in potassium for good health. Most processed foods use sodium so if you stick to whole, less processed foods you'll naturally lower the sodium in your diet.

High Energy Foods

The best choices for energizing foods are the ones that are rich in carbohydrates. Put these foods together along with low fat protein and high fiber foods for energy throughout the day.

Omega 3 Fatty Acid Rich Foods

- Mackeral
- Sardines
- Albacore tuna
- Walnuts
- Flaxseed
- Conola oil
- Soy beans (soy milk)
- Cereals
- Omega-3 fortified foods

High Energy Foods

- Sweet potatoes
- Tomatoes
- 100% fruit juices
- 100% vegetable juices
- Blueberries
- Cantalope
- Cirtus fruit
- Mangoes
- Strawberries
- Most whole fruits
- Dried fruits
- Nuts
- Beans
- Low fat dairy products
- Whole grains

Best to Buy Organic

The nonprofit Environmental Working Group says these 12 are among the most susceptible to pesticide residue. Buy these foods organic whenever possible.

SOURCE: Kathleen Zelman, MPH, RD, LD, Director of Nutrition for WebMD.

High Potassium

- Mushrooms
- Peas
- Potatoes
- Spinach
- Sweet potatoes
- Tomatoes
- Bananas
- Grapefruit
- Oranges
- Beans
- Lentils
- Low fat or fat free dairy
- Raisins
- Kiwi

Best to Buy Organic

- Celery
- Lettuce
- Potatoes
- Spinach
- Sweet bell peppers
- Apples
- Cherries
- Grapes (imported)
- Peaches
- Pears
- Nectarines
- Strawberries

Today's Challenge

Today I challenge you to become a conscious eater. When you go to the grocery store look for foods on the Healthy Foods list and add them to the cart. Read labels, choose more organic foods when possible and make a decision today to eat to live, not live to eat.

Day 21 Affirmation

"Be anxious for nothing, but in everything by prayer and supplication, with thanksgiving, let your requests be made known to God."

Philippians 4:6

WHAT DID YOU LEARN FROM TODAY'S READING AND WHAT DID YOU LEARN ABOUT YOURSELF?

_____
_____
_____
_____
_____
_____
_____
_____
_____
_____
_____

HOW WILL YOU TAKE ONE STEP TOWARDS LIVING A HEALTHIER LIFESTYLE TODAY?

_____
_____
_____
_____
_____
_____
_____
_____
_____
_____
_____

LIST THREE THINGS (ANY THING)YOU'RE PROUD OF
YOURSELF FOR TODAY AND EXPLAIN WHY:

_____

_____

_____

_____

_____

_____

_____

_____

_____

_____

_____

_____

_____

_____

_____

_____

SPEND FIVE MINUTES TODAY RECONNECTING YOUR
SPIRIT TO GOD. WRITE IT, PRAY IT OR SHOW IT!

_____

_____

_____

_____

_____

_____

_____

_____

_____

_____

_____

_____

_____

_____

_____

_____

Epilogue

The Chinese philosopher Lao-tzu said, "A journey of a thousand miles begins with a single step." Take a moment and think about the journey you've just begun. You took the first step when you made the decision to take back your body and live a healthier lifestyle. For whatever reason, something inside of you finally woke up and said, "Enough!" No more sabotaging your health, no more excuses about exercise, and no more mindless eating. You realized that you deserve better and were willing to step out on faith and make it happen. I'm so proud of you! It takes strength and courage to recognize your own faults and then do something about them. The simple lifestyle changes you've learned in this book will help you achieve your goal of better health and fitness, and I can't wait to hear about it!

I want you to continue to practice what you've learned in this book and use the Affirmation pages to motivate you through the rough spots. You wrote them and nobody knows how your mind works better than you! Learn from them, recognize the pitfalls that have held you back and vow to release yourself from them forever. Lao-tzu didn't say anything about the journey being easy; he said it begins with a single step. Use the tools in this book to help guide you, strengthen you and most of all know that you're not alone on this journey; God is with you every step of the way.

Join me and countless other women as we continue the revolution online at, SweetTeaRevolution.com. Become a member, share your stories and join me and other women for laid back, frank discussions about the issues that are important to us as black women today. You can also follow me on Twitter @SweetTeaRev when you need a laugh, kick in the butt or pat on the back. We're all in this together and when two or more agree, the Lord said it shall be done!

I'm going to leave you now with a poem written especially for this book by a very close friend of mine. She took the essence of Sweet Tea and Cornbread and created a work of art. Much love and success to you all. Enjoy!

Sweet Tea & Cornbread

By Constance Bones

Mmmmm!

Sweet tea and cornbread! Oooh, on a hot summa's day.
How does that sound, with you and ya girls sittin' around?
Takin' in the summa's rays and talkin' bout black folk's
ways;
Sippin' on sweet tea, and nibblin' on cornbread!
Yep... that's what I said.

Honey chile, yeah... I'm talkin' to you... care for some
sweet tea and cornbread?
Just a snack to carry you thru... till the evening spread.

Black women's roots run deep down in the South,
We'z blessed with exquisite taste, and a sassy mouth.
At an early age, we'z taught the true meanin' of sweet tea
and cornbread.

Honey chile, yeah... I'm talkin' to you... care for some
sweet tea and cornbread?
Just a snack to carry you thru... till the evening spread.

A Southern life style ain't no ordinary life,
It's about creatin' memories of love, and livin' thru the
strife.
Chit chattin' on the outdoor stoop,
Discussin' who is in...or out the loop.
Watchin' dark, sexy, sweaty brotha's shootin' hoop.
Young girls twistin', movin' and singin' to the latest beat.
Babies...and daddies maybe,
Beatin' the summa's heat.
The occasional lust gone too far,
Youngster profilin' in da family car.

And through it all ...Southerner's love to praise the Lawd!
Reminiscin' bout the dead, drink sweet tea by the gallons,
And nibble on fresh hot cornbread.
Yep... that's what I said.

Honey chile, yeah... I'm talkin' to you... care for some
sweet tea and cornbread?
Just a snack to carry you thru... till the evening spread.

Resources

I thought it would be helpful to include a few of my favorite resources, apps and websites to keep your mind on your health and your health on your mind.

Websites

heart.org – The American Heart Association
americanlungassociation.org – The American Lung Association
diabetes.org – American Diabetes Association
fnic.nal.usda.gov – United States Department of Agriculture
cdc.gov – Centers for Disease Control and Prevention
webmd.com – Medical advice, health information and resources
mayoclinic.com – Medical advice, health information and research
oldwayspt.org – Nutrition information through heritage
livestrong.com – General health information

Apps

My Fitness Pal – Calorie and exercise counter (ipad, iphone) Free!
Food Meter – Calorie scanner (ipad, iphone) Free!
Run Keeper – GPS and tracker for running, walking, etc (ipad, iphone) Free!
Lose It – Calorie and exercise counter (for Nook) Free!
Daily Arm, Leg, Butt, Ab, Cardio Workouts (for Nook) $0.99ea
Grocery Shopping List (for Nook) $0.99

Healthy Recipe Websites

Foodnetwork.com
Epicurious.com
Eatingwell.com
Myrecipes.com
Oldwayspt.org
Mayoclinic.com/health/healthy-recipes/RecipeIndex (Great for chronic disease related recipes like the DASH diet)

Endnotes

[1] Workout for Endomorphs | Exercise for Endomorphs, http://www.superskinnyme.com/endomorph-workout-plan.html (accessed May 22, 2012).

[2] Quiz: Do You Know the Difference Between Salt and Sodium? http://www.healthcentral.com/high-blood-pressure/lifestyle-270673.html (accessed may 22, 2012).

[3] High Blood Pressure and African Americans, http://www.amhrt.org/HEARTORG/Conditions/HighBloodPressure/Understanding YourRiskforHighBloodPressure/High-Blood-Pressure-and-African-Americans_UCM_301832_Artical.jsp (accessed May 22, 2012).

[4] Tips for Reducing Sodium in Your Diet – NIH Heart, Lung and…, http://www.nhlbi.nih.gov/hbp/prevent/sodium/tips/htm (accessed May 22, 2012)

[5] White Bread vs. Wheat Bread | Vegetarian Times, http://www.vegetariantimes.com/article/white-bread-vs-wheat-bread/ (accessed May 22, 2012).

[6] Good Carbs vs. Bad Carbs | http://www.everydayhealth.com/diet-nutrition/101/nutrition-basics/good-carbs-bad-carbs.aspx (accessed May 22, 2012).

[7] List of Foods in the Grain Group | LIVESTONG.COM, http://www.livestong.com/article/84874-list-foods-grain-group/ (accessed May 22, 2012).

[8] Healthy Soul Food Menus | LIVESTRONG.COM, http://www.livestong.com/srticle/275910-healthy-soul-food-menus/ (accessed May 22, 2012).

[9] Caring for Your Health | MyFoodPyramid.gov/Pyramid/Vegetables.html (accessed May, 22, 21012).

[10] Caring for Your Health | MyFoodPyramid.gov/Pyramid/Grains.html (accessed May, 22, 21012).

[11] On The Move to Better Heart Health for African Americans | http://www.nhlbi.nih.gov/health/public/heart/other/chdblack/ (accessed May 22, 1012).

[12] Not So Sweet – The Average American Consumes 150-170 Pounds…, http://sites.google.com/site/thehealthinfosite/home/nutrition/not-so-sweet---the-average-american-consumes-150-170-pounds-of-sugar-each-year (accessed May 22, 2012).

[13] Foods Low In Refined Sugars | LIVESTONG.COM, http://www.livestong.com/article/81991-foods-low-refined-sugars/ (accessed May 22, 2012).

[14] Sugars and Carbohydrates, http://www.heart.ort/HEARTORG/GettingHealthy/NutritionCenter/HealthyDietG oals/Sugars-and-Carbohydrates_UCM_303296-Articla.JSP (accessed May 22, 2012).

[15] Artificial sweetners: Understanding these and other sugar…, http://www.mayoclinic.com/health/artifical-sweetners/MY00073 (accessed May 22, 1012)

[16] The Epi-Log on Epicurious.com: Sugar News—and It's Not Good, http://www.epicurious.com/features_editor/2011/05/sugar-news-and-its-not-good.html (accessed May 22, 2012).

[17] The Fat In Fried Foods | LIVESTONG.COM,http://www.livestrong.com/article/460878-the-fat-in-fried-food/(accessed May 23, 2012).

[18] Dietary Fats: What Type To Choose, http://www.mayoclinic.com/health/fat/NU00262 (accessed May 23, 2012).

[19] Tips For Choosing The Best Types Of Fat, http://www.mayoclinic.com/health/fat/NU00262/NSECTIONGROUP=2 (accessed May 23, 2012).

[20] How To Reduce Your Risk | http://www.cnpp.usda.gov/Publications/DietaryGuidelines/2010/PolicyDoc/PolicyDoc.pdf (accessed May, 22,2012).

[21] Why Portion Sizes Are Important, http://healthlibrary.brighamanwomens.org/Library/Wellness/1,2015 (accessed May 23, 2012

[22] Does Not Eating After A Certain Time Help You Lose Weight…,http://www.livestrong.com/article/533820-does-not-eating-after-a-certain-time-help-you-lose-weight/ (accessed May 23, 2012).

[23] Snack Attack! – WebMD – Better Information, Better Health, http://www.webmd.com/diet/features/snack-attack (accessed May 23, 2012).

[24] How ManyFruits And Vegebales Do You Need | http://www.fruitsandveggiesmatter.gov/downloads/General_Audience_Brochure.pdf (accessed May 22, 2012).

[25] Metabolism and weight loss: How you burn calories.., http://www.mayoclinic.com/health/metabolism/WT00006 (accessed May 23, 2012).

[26] Metabolism and weight loss: How you burn calories…, http://www.mayoclinic.com/health/metabolis/WT00006/NSECTIONGROUP=2 (accessed May 23, 2012).

[27] Five Most Important Recommended Supplements: http://www.realage.com/blogs/doctor-oz-roizen/5-most-important-recommended-supplements (accessed Jun 11, 2012)

[28] Reading Food Nutrition Labels: http://www.heart.org/HEARTORG/GettingHealthy/NutritionCenter/HeartSmartShopping/Reading-Food-Nutrition-Labels_UCM_300132_Article.jsp (accessed May 30, 2012)

[29] How to Read a Nutrition Label – WebMD- Better Information…,http://www.webmd.com/food-recipes/features/how-to-read-nutrition-label (accessed May 23, 2012).